The
ANTIHISTAMINE DIET

COOKBOOK WITH DELICIOUS, NOURISHING, LOW-HISTAMINE RECIPES

Greta Pitts

TABLE OF CONTENTS

INTRODUCTION

If you bought the book because you are histamine intolerant or have an unconfirmed suspicion of being histamine intolerant, you deal with symptoms that are anything but pleasant.

Histamine is an amino acid found in food and is produced as a waste product by microorganisms. Still, histamine is also produced naturally in your body because it has specific functions to do.

Our eating habits, in particular, have a significant influence, and diet plays an essential role in histamine intolerance because, with exceptional nutrition care, you can improve your daily well-being.

If you suffer from histamine intolerance, you should always pay attention to the following rules:

- Food should be prepared and consumed as fresh as possible;

- Fermented foods, which are also lactic acids, should disappear from your menu, such as sauerkraut;

- Certain types of fish such as mackerel, anchovy, herring, and tuna should be avoided;

- you should prefer frozen products;

- Fish should always be soaked in water before preparation and processing; this reduces the histamine content;

- you should also avoid alcoholic beverages;

- Only short-aged cheeses should end up on your plates, such as butter cheese, young Gouda, or cream cheese;

- In the case of cheese, you should permanently remove the rind generously;

- you should avoid smoked or long-aged sausages. Use, for

example, cooked ham instead;

- Sweets should generally be reduced or omitted;
- Preserved foods and prepared meals should be avoided;
- Always process or enjoy well-chilled foods;
- Pay attention to the proper cold chain. If frozen goods have burned or ice crystals have formed on the product, it is best not to consume it.

There has probably been an error in the cold chain, so you cannot rule out an increase or high histamine content.

In addition to these rules, I would like to present the foods that you should avoid and that you are allowed to eat. Often you leave out parts of different foods, and you will soon feel better. You will then find a table with categories of tolerable, unsafe, or incompatible foods. Dangerous foods, in this case, mean that some people can tolerate them despite histamine intolerance. On the other hand, people cannot accept them, and symptoms develop. So you will need to test these foods to see if they are suitable for you or not.

MEAT AND EGGS

Compatible: Fresh and natural meat, Frozen meat (quickly thawed and prepared, Boiled Ham, Eggs

Unsure: Fresh Meat from the open market, Packaged minced meat, Cooled sausage and fresh sausage, Game Meat

Incompatible: Canned Meat (cured, marinated, smoked, atc...), Dried Meat, Raw Ham, Grisons Meat, Bacon, Meat that has matured on the bone or hung for a long time, Chopped or pureed meat products (meat loaf, liver sausage, etc.), Offal, All sausage products such as salami, bratwurst, cervelat etc.

FISH AND SEAFOOD

Compatible: Freshly caught fish directly from the fisherman or breeding station, Frozen fish (thawed and prepared directly).

Unsure: Fish from the fresh food counter, market stall or restaurant, Seafood.

Incompatible: Canned fish, Marinated, salted, dried or smoked fish, Pickled fish, Tuna, mackerel, herring, sardines, anchovies and mahi mahi, Mussels, crabs, prawns, lobsters, and shrimp, other crustaceans

MILK AND MILK PRODUCTS

Compatible: Fresh milk straight from the cow, UHT milk or pasteurized milk, Butter, cream, cream and whey, Fresh cheese and milk products such as mozzarella, mascarpone, quark, young Gouda cheese and butter cheese

Unsure: Feta cheese, yogurt and kefir, sour milk, such as buttermilk, sour cream, etc.

Incompatible: matured cheeses, such as hard cheese, Semi-hard cheese, soft cheese, processed cheese, blue cheese, old Gouda and Fondue cheese.

CEREALS, BAKED GOODS AND STARCHY PRODUCTS

Compatible: potatoes, rice and corn, grains, meal, semolina, flour and baked goods of this kind.

Unsure: Malt, Wheat Germs, Canned Corn, Unpeeled Buckwheat.

Incompatible: yeast and sourdough, Very Fresh, still warm backed goods.

VEGETABLES AND MUSHROOMS

Compatible: All types, except for those who are "incompatible" in the category are found.

Unsure: Green French beans, Peas, Olives that do not undergo lactic acid fermentation were subjected, Mushrooms.

Incompatible: Sauerkraut, Spinach, Tomatoes and their products (ketchup etc...), Legumes, Soy Products, Pickled Foods, porcini Mushrooms, Morels and Mushrooms.

OILS AND FATS

Compatible: Vegetable Oils, Vegetable fats, Animal Fats, Fish Oil

Unsure: Walnut Oil

Incompatible: None in this category

FISH AND SEAFOOD

Compatible: Table Salt, Garlic, Kitchen Herbs fresh and dried, Mild Spices, alcohol Vinegar, Brandy Vinegar, Apple Cider, Vinegar and Vinegar Essence, Corn Starch, Potato Starch.

Unsure: None in this category.

Incompatible: Wine Vinegar, Balsamic Vinegar, Yeast Extracts, Flavor enhancers such as glutamate, Sodium glutamate, Boullion and Broth, Soy Sauce, Hot Spices.

SWEETS AND SWEETENERS

Compatible: Sugar, Agave Syrup, Honey, Stevia, Jam made from the compatible fruits.

Unsure: White Chocolate.

Incompatible: Cocoa, Cocoa Mass, Brown and dark Chocolate, Carob.

BEVERAGES

Compatible: Water, Herbal tea, Natural rooibos, Juice and Fruit nectars, lemonade if compatible ingredients, Almond Milk.

Unsure: Rice Milk, Oat Milk, Spirits (clear), Espresso, Black tea, Green tea, Coffee.

Incompatible: Alcohol, Soy Milk, Energy Drinks, Juices and

Lemonades with incompatible ingredients, Nettle Tea.

FRUITS, SEEDS AND NUTS

Compatible: All varieties, except those that can be found in the "incompatible" category

Unsure: Overripe fruit, Fruit with rotten spots

Incompatible: Strawberry, Raspberry, Citrus Fruits, Bananas, Kiwi, Pears, papaya, Guava, Walnuts, Cashews, Peanuts

Below I present you some low histamine recipes to offer you the most incredible possible variety of culinary dishes every day.

Nutritional plans are a great help when they are set up correctly, but a health plan is only good if it is adapted to your needs, so among these recipes, you will have to choose the most compatible with your body.

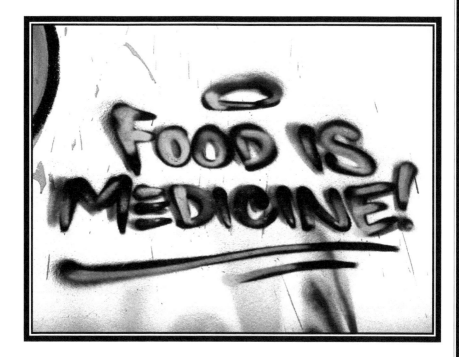

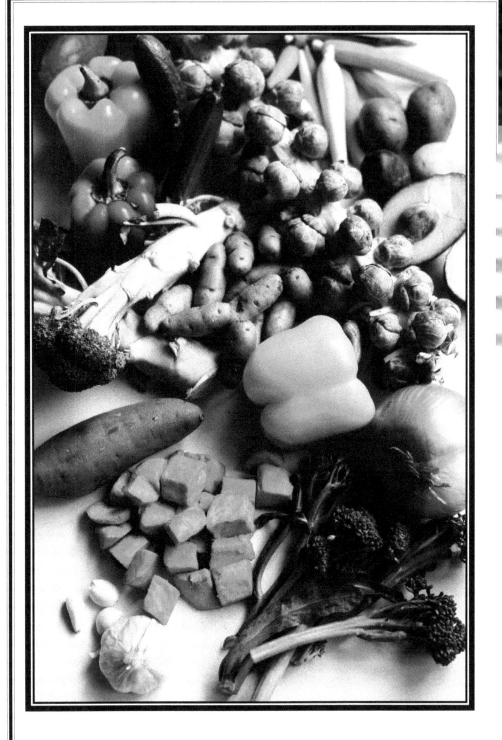

BREAKFAST

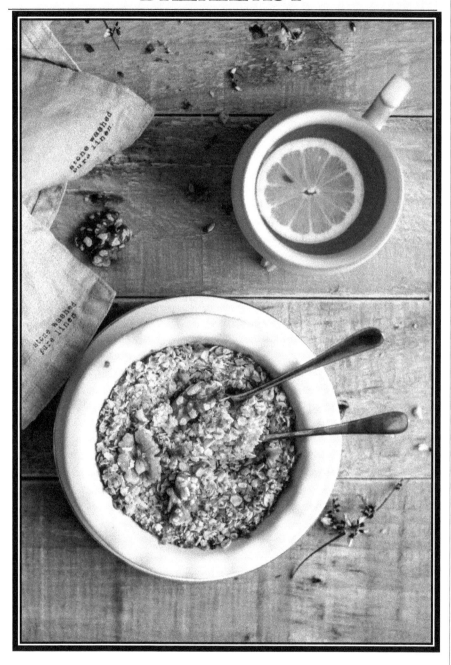

1.Coconut semolina

Direction time: 15 minutes
Servings: 2 servings
Difficulty level: Very easy

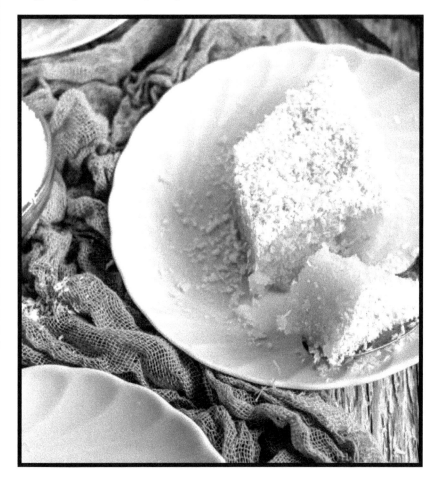

Nutritional information
Kcal 144; protein 5g; fat 2g; carbohydrates 26g

INGREDIENTS

- **50** G SPELLED SEMOLINA
- **SOME** BUTTER
- **40** G OF GLUCOSE
- **500** ML COCONUT MILK
- **1** PINCH OF SALT
- **4** TBSP COCONUT FLAKES
- **SOME** CINNAMON TO SPRINKLE

DIRECTIONS

1. Warm the milk in a saucepan and stir in the salt, rice syrup (if using household sugar or honey, only use 30 g) and butter.

2. As soon as the milk is heated, add the semolina and stir well until everything is completely dissolved. Cook the mixture over high heat, stirring constantly, until it becomes thicker. Then reduce the temperature, add the coconut flakes and let everything simmer for a few minutes.

3. As soon as the mass no longer drips from the spoon, it is done.

4. Put the semolina in suitable bowls and serve. If necessary, the semolina can be garnished with desiccated coconut.

2. SPELLED PORRIDGE

Direction time: 15 minutes
Servings: 2 servings
Difficulty level: Very easy

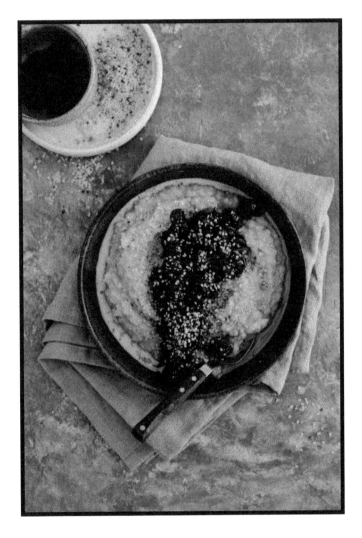

Nutritional information
Kcal 134; protein 4 g; fat 2 g; carbohydrates 23 g

INGREDIENTS

- **85** G SPELLED FLAKES
- **200 - 250** ML UNSWEETENED
- **ALMOND MILK**
- **1** TBSP HONEY
- **2** TEASPOONS OF GROUND MEAT LINSEED
- **2** TEASPOONS OF CHIA SEEDS
- **50** G BLUEBERRIES
- **1** APRICOT
- **50** G PEACH

DIRECTIONS

1. Firstly, mix the oat flakes well with the liquid of your choice and simmer everything over low heat for about 5-10.

2. Add the chia seeds and the flax seeds.

3. Wash and chop the fruit well and garnish on the porridge.

4. Finally, let some honey drip onto the porridge and enjoy warm.

NOTE

The honey can easily be replaced with rice syrup and the vegetable milk with water or other vegetable milk.

3.SWEET CORN COOK

Direction time: 15 minutes
Servings: 4 servings
Difficulty level: Very easy

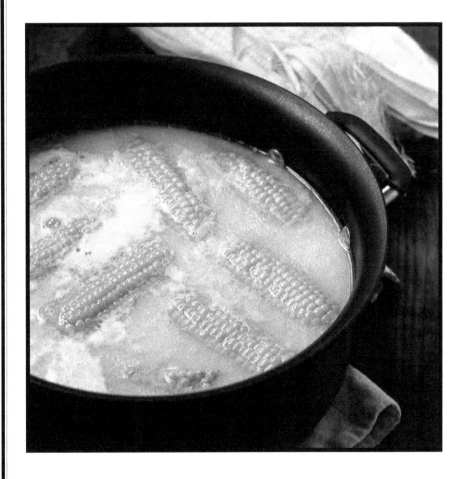

Nutritional information
Kcal 233; protein 8 g; fat 4 g; carbohydrates 31 g

INGREDIENTS

- **10** G BUTTER
- **1.5** L UNSWEETENED ALMOND MILK
- **500** ML OF WATER
- **160** G POLENTA / CORN GRITS
- **1** PINCH OF SALT
- SOME CINNAMON OF YOUR OWN TASTE
- SOME HONEY OF YOUR OWN
- SWEET TASTE
- BLUEBERRIES, OR PEACHES
- OTHER WHOLESOME FRUIT

DIRECTIONS

1. Heat the butter in a pan with a high rim.
2. Add milk and bring carefully to the boil.
3. Mix the corn flour with the water and let it boil down while stirring constantly. A good tasting crust is created on the bottom, which is called "Prinze" in Tyrol. Then take the pan off the heat, add the fruit and stir well. Finally, sweeten everything with cinnamon and sugar or sweeteners and enjoy.

NOTE:

If it lumps - you haven't stirred enough, but that doesn't matter. Puree the mixture once before you add the fruit and your chef will taste delicately creamy.

4. COFFEE GRANOLA

Direction time: 30 minutes
Servings: 350 g
Difficulty level: Very easy

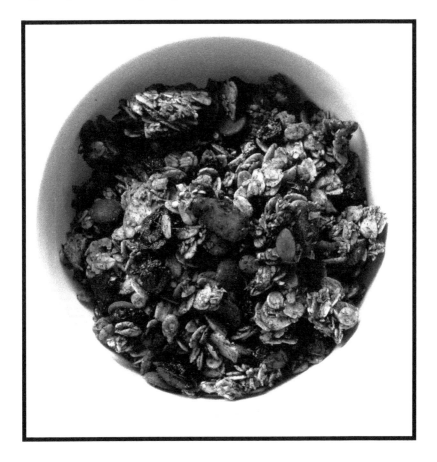

Nutritional information
Kcal 276; protein 6 g; fat 19 g; carbohydrates 33 g

INGREDIENTS

- **250** G **5-GRAIN FLAKES, ALTERNATIVELY OAT FLAKES**
- **50** G OF OAT BRAN
- **2** TBSP RAPE SEED OIL
- **6** TBSP COLD ESPRESSO
- **2** TBSP SUGAR BEET SYRUP
- **1** TBSP RAW CANE SUGAR
- **100** G WHITE CHOCOLATE

DIRECTIONS

1. Firstly, put the flakes with the oat bran in a bowl and mix well.

2. Boil the espresso and let it cool completely. Then mix well with the rapeseed oil, sugar beet syrup and raw cane sugar.

3. Now pour everything over the flakes and mix well too.

4. Preheat the oven to 175 degrees and line a baking sheet with parchment paper. Spread the mixture well over it. Now bake everything for about 15-20 minutes and then let it cool down well.

5. Portion the muesli as desired and enjoy.

NOTE:

Not everyone can handle espresso or white chocolate. Therefore, please approach the recipe carefully! If necessary, omit the white chocolate or espresso. If the muesli is packaged airtight, it will keep for up to four weeks. To cool the muesli faster, you can put cold towels under the baking sheet and cool it down faster. However, the cloths have to be changed regularly.

5. BIRCHER MUESLI

Direction time: 20 minutes
Servings: 2 servings
Difficulty level: Very easy

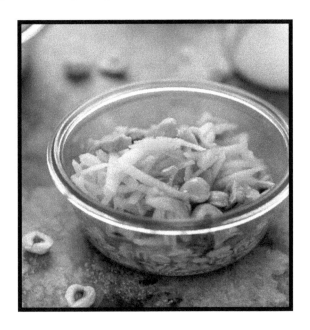

INGREDIENTS

- **80** G OAT FLAKES
- **30** G RAISINS
- **125** ML APPLE JUICE
- **30** G COMPATIBLE NUTS (OPTIONAL)
- **200** G APPLE, GRATED
- **120** G GRAPES
- **250** G YOGURT, ALTERNATIVELY
- CREAM CHEESE

- SOME HONEY FOR SWEETENING
- 50 G BLUEBERRIES
- 1 TEASPOON CHIA SEEDS
- 1 TBSP PUMPKIN SEEDS
- 2 TEASPOONS OF FLAXSEED

DIRECTIONS

1. Mix raisins, cereal flakes (coarse or fine-leaved), coarsely chopped nuts and apple juice in a bowl and steep or swell overnight.

2. The next day: Wash the apples well and grate them using a kitchen grater. If necessary, the apple can be peeled and drizzled with lemon juice so that it does not turn brown - but neither is necessary (peel and drizzle).

3. Then clean the grapes cut them in two and remove the seeds if necessary.

4. Finally, mix the mixture well with the yoghurt and sour cream and serve in suitable bowls.

NOTE:

The muesli can be wonderfully refined with different fruits, such as blueberries, peaches, flax seeds, pumpkin seeds, sunflower seeds and much more. The muesli also tastes very good with Greek yoghurt - but it is then very rich, as the fat content is higher than with normal yoghurt. If the Bircher muesli is too firm, just add a little more milk / vegetable milk or yoghurt / cream cheese.

Nutritional information
Kcal 254; protein 7 g; fat 10 g; carbohydrates 26 g

6.RHUBARB JELLY

Direction time: 90 minutes
Servings: 5 glasses of 230 ml capacity each capital
Difficulty level: Very easy

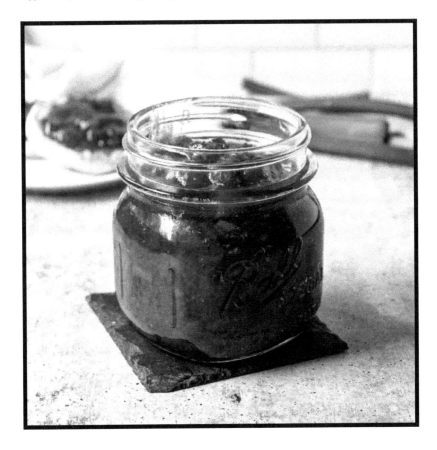

Nutritional information
Kcal 438; protein 2 g; fat 0 g; carbohydrates 104 g

INGREDIENTS

- **1.5** KG OF RHUBARB
- **20** G VANILLA SUGAR
- **500** G PRESERVING SUGAR **2: 1** WITHOUT LEMON JUICE OR ACID ARE AVAILABLE IN HEALTH FOOD STORES

DIRECTIONS

1. First peel the rhubarb and cut into small pieces.
2. Put 500ml of water, the vanilla sugar and the rhubarb in a saucepan. Let everything simmer for about 10 minutes over medium heat.
3. Place a kitchen towel in a colander and place over a bowl. Put the soft boiled rhubarb with juice in the kitchen towel and let drip for about 60 minutes.
4. Measure 750ml of the juice. You can drink the rest of the mixture as a spritzer mixed with water.
5. Cook the rhubarb juice with the preserving sugar according to the instructions on the packet.
6. Tip into jam jars and close immediately.
7. Store the cooled glasses in a cool, dry place.

NOTE :

If the draining time seems too long, you can also buy directly pressed rhubarb juice. But make sure that the rhubarb juice is natural and untreated and consists of 100% rhubarb.

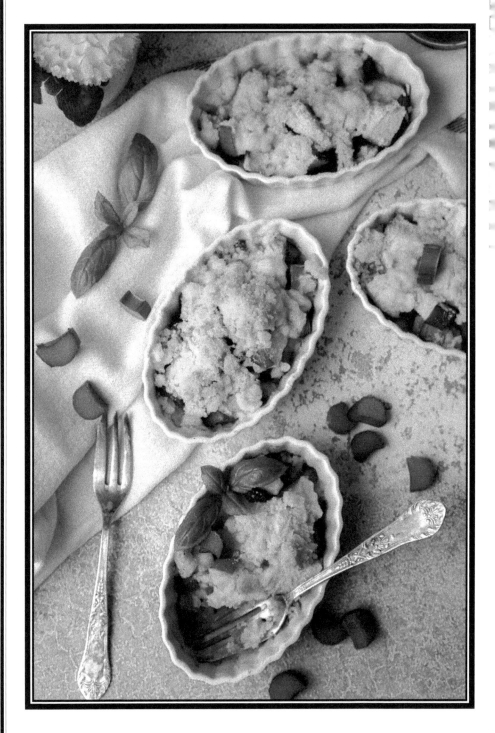

LUNCH

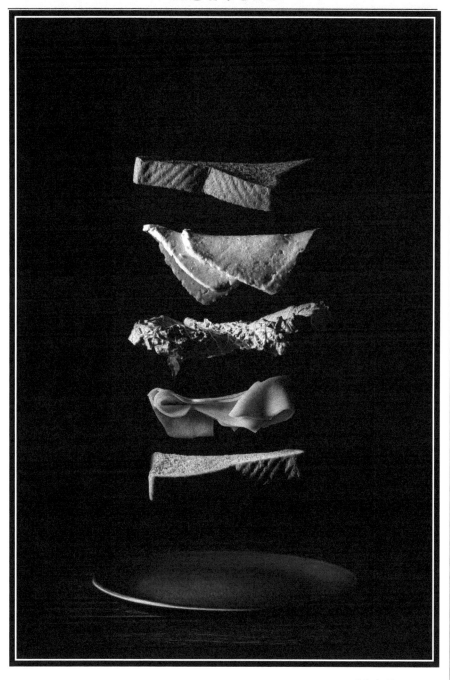

7.PANGASIUS FILLET IN CORN BREADING WITH RICE

Direction time: 35 minutes
Servings: 2 servings
Difficulty level: normal

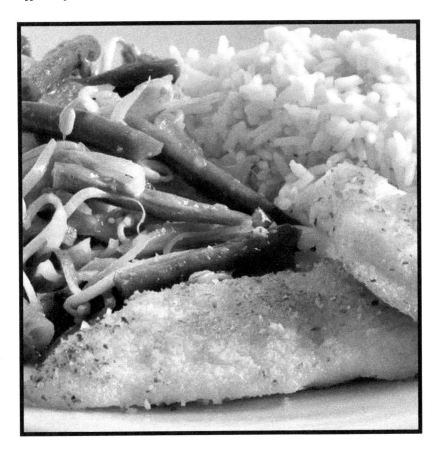

Nutritional information
Kcal 501; protein 39 g; fat 15 g; carbohydrates 51 g

INGREDIENTS

- **400** G PANGASIUS FILLET , FROZEN, FRESHLY PROCESSED
- **125** G BASMATI RICE
- **1** CARROT
- **100** G CORN FLOUR
- **70** G CORN FLAKES, UNSWEETENED
- **2** EGG YOLKS
- DILL, TO TASTE
- SALT
- OIL, FOR FRYING

DIRECTIONS

1. Thaw the pangasius fillet quickly (preferably in the microwave) so that no histamine forms. Rinse the fillets briefly and pat dry. Add dill, salt and, if you like, pepper (be careful with histamine intolerance, not everyone can tolerate pepper).

2. Now first turn the fillets in the corn flour, then pull them through the whisked egg yolk, finally bread with the coarsely crumbled corn flakes and press everything down well.

3. Let some oil get hot in the pan and fry the fillets on both sides until golden brown for about ten minutes.

4. In the meantime, bring 2 large glasses of water with salt to the boil and add the rice.

5. Chop the carrots and add them to the rice with the saucepan. Cook over medium heat until the rice is cooked through and the water has been absorbed by the rice. Arrange the vegetable rice together with the fish on plates and serve immediately.

8.ZUCCHINI RICOTTA RISOTTO

Direction time: 30 minutes
Servings: 4 servings
Difficulty level: Easy

INGREDIENTS

- **400** G RISOTTO RICE
- **200** G RICOTTA
- **2** MEDIUM ZUCCHINI
- **1** RED ONION
- **2** TBSP OLIVE OIL
- **1** L VEGETABLE STOCK

DIRECTIONS

1. Peel the onion and cut into fine cubes.

2. Let the oil get hot in a pan. Sweat the onions and rice in them until translucent for 1-2 minutes, add the zucchini and let them sweat briefly. Pour a little broth over everything and let it boil over low heat, mixing regularly.

3. When the liquid is absorbed, add gradually the rest of the stock, stirring occasionally. Cook for about 20 minutes, until the rice is soft but still has a bit of bite. Finally, work in the ricotta and serve hot immediately.

Nutritional information
Kcal 267; protein 11 g; fat 9 g; carbohydrates 31 g

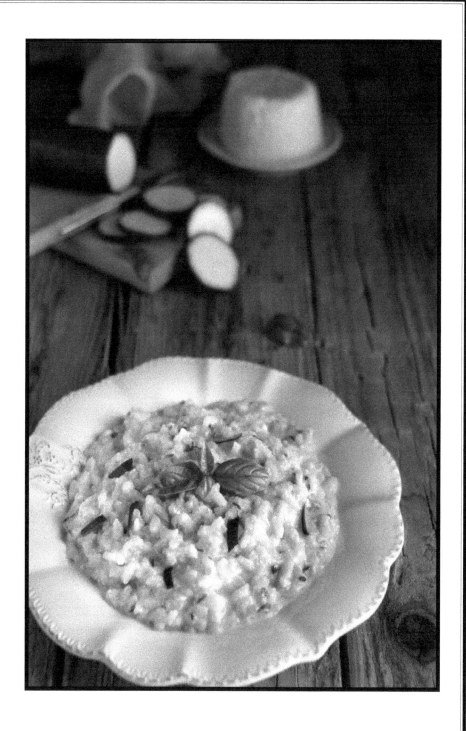

9.MINCED PATTIES FROM THE OVEN

Direction time: 45 minutes
Servings: 4 servings
Difficulty level: Easy

INGREDIENTS

- **1** KG MINCED BEEF (FRESH AND SELF-MINCED)
- **8** TEASPOONS OF POTATO STARCH OR OTHER STARCH
- **8** TBSP MINERAL WATER WITH
- CARBONIC ACID
- **4** TBSP POTATO FLAKES (POTATO FLAKES FROM A PACK FOR MASHED POTATOES), LOW IN HISTAMINE, WITHOUT ADDITIVES
- **4** TBSP PARSLEY, FINELY CHOPPED
- SOME BUTTER
- N.B. SALT AND PEPPER
- N.B. SOUP SPICE , GLUTEN-FREE AND LOW IN HISTAMINE (E.G. HILDEGARD VON BINGEN SOUP SPICE)

DIRECTIONS

1. Mix the potato starch with the sparkling water in a large bowl. Then mix with the rest of the ingredients and knead well. Divide into portions and firmly shape by hand.

2. Bake on a baking sheet lined with baking paper in the preheated oven at 180 degrees for about 30 minutes on the middle rack, until the dish is cooked through. Let cool down briefly and serve immediately.

Nutritional information
Kcal 430; protein 15 g; fat 17 g; carbohydrates 28 g

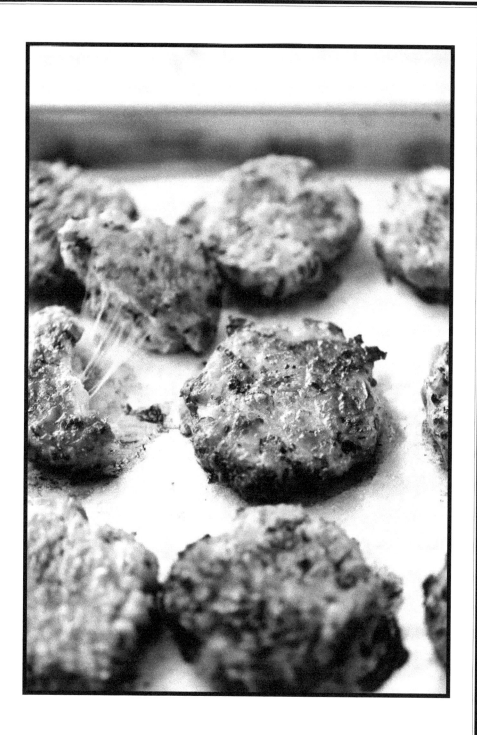

10. POULTRY WITH STEWED VEGETABLES

Direction time: 25 minutes
Servings: 1 serving
Difficulty level: normal

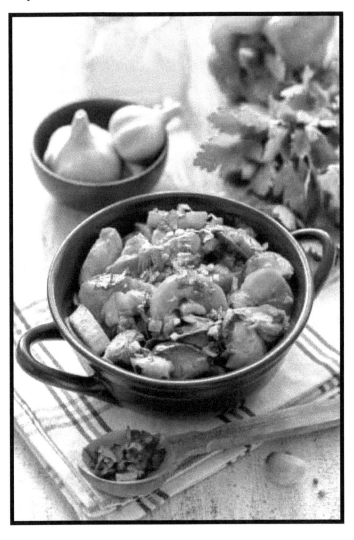

INGREDIENTS

- **180** G CHICKEN (BREAST)
- **250** G POTATOES
- **1** ZUCCHINI
- **2** SHALLOTS (APPROX. 30 G)
- **150** G CARROT
- **1** CLOVE OF GARLIC
- **1** PINCH OF IODIZED SALT
- **1** PINCH OF PEPPER (BLACK)
- **1** PINCH OF HERBS (FROZEN, ITALIAN)
- **1** TBSP OLIVE OIL

DIRECTIONS

1. Bring the oven to 200 degrees.

2. Peel the skin of the potatoes, cut into wedges and mix with a little oil and spices in a bowl.

3. Spread on a baking sheet lined with baking paper and bake in a preheated oven at 200 degrees for around 20 minutes until golden brown.

4. In the meantime, fry the chicken until golden brown and cut the vegetables into cubes.

5. Cook the vegetables with a little oil in a closed saucepan over a low heat for about 10 minutes and season with spices at the end. Arrange the vegetables with the chicken on plates and serve immediately.

Nutritional information
Kcal 274; protein 5 g; fat 10 g; carbohydrates 31 g

11. KOHLRABI CHICKEN RAGOUT

Direction time: 30 minutes
Servings: 1 serving
Difficulty level: normal

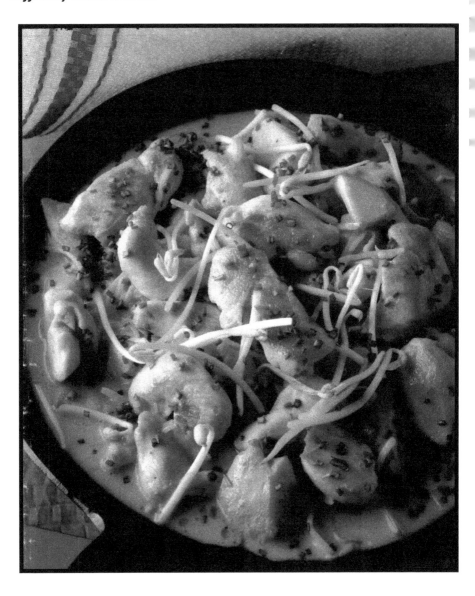

INGREDIENTS

- **125** G CHICKEN (BREAST)
- **½** KOHLRABI
- **½** ONION
- **30** ML MILK (LOW-FAT **1.5%** FAT)
- **30** ML CRÈME LÉGÈRE
- **½** TSP VEGETABLE STOCK
- **¼** BUNCH OF PARSLEY
- **2** TEASPOONS OF OLIVE OIL

DIRECTIONS

1. Cut the meat and kohlrabi into cubes.
2. Salt and pepper the diced meat and fry in oil. Then keep the meat warm.
3. In the same pan, sauté the onion cubes and pour in the milk, then add the kohlrabi to the pan and add 50 ml of stock.
4. Cook with the lid on for 15 minutes.
5. Put the crème légère and chicken back in the pan and bring everything to the boil again.
6. Season with salt, pepper and nutmeg.
7. Scatter finely chopped parsley over the dish to serve.

Nutritional information
446 kcal; protein 33 g; fat 21 g; carbohydrates 39 g

12. FAR EASTERN CHICKEN IN COCONUT SAUCE

Direction time: 75 minutes
Servings: 3 servings
Difficulty level: normal

INGREDIENTS

- **500** G CORN-FED CHICKEN BREAST FILLET
- **1** RED PEPPER
- **1** ZUCCHINI
- **2** CARROTS
- **200** ML VEGETABLE STOCK, HOT, FREE OF YEAST AND SOY
- **300** ML COCONUT MILK, CREAMY
- **1** HEAPED TEASPOON CORN STARCH, GLUTEN FREE
- **2** TEASPOONS OF COCONUT OIL
- **1** BUNCH OF CHIVES
- **1** TEASPOON PAPRIKA POWDER, NOBLE SWEET
- **1** LEVEL TEASPOON SALT
- **2** PINCHES OF PEPPER
- **300** G RICE

DIRECTIONS

1. Wash the vegetables and chives thoroughly.
2. Peel the skin of the carrots and cut into thin slices. Cut the peppers into pieces. Cut the zucchini lengthways and cut into slices. Cut the chives into fine rolls.

3. Wash the chicken fillet, pat dry with kitchen paper and cut into cubes.

4. For the rice, put water in a saucepan, season with salt and bring to a boil. Now prepare the rice according to the instructions on the packet.

5. Heat 2 teaspoons of coconut oil in a pan. Fry the chicken cubes in coconut oil, then add the vegetables and fry briefly. Season to taste with salt and paprika. Pour in the hot vegetable stock, shortly afterwards stir in the coconut milk and let it simmer for about 10-15 minutes.

6. Thicken the sauce with the cornstarch. Mix 2 level teaspoons of cornstarch with a little cold water until smooth, add to the sauce and bring to the boil while stirring. Finally, work in the fresh chives and season again with salt and pepper.

7. Serve with the rice.

TIP :

Beware of histamine intolerance - the vegetable broth should be free from yeast and soy!

Paprika, zucchini and carrots are low-histamine vegetables. Coconut milk is free from histamine, lactose and gluten.

Nutritional information
505 kcal; protein 41 g; fat 14 g; carbohydrates 51 g

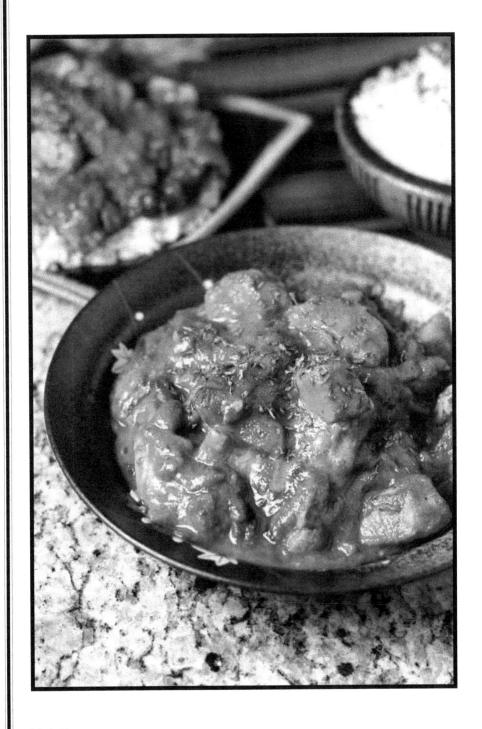

DINNER

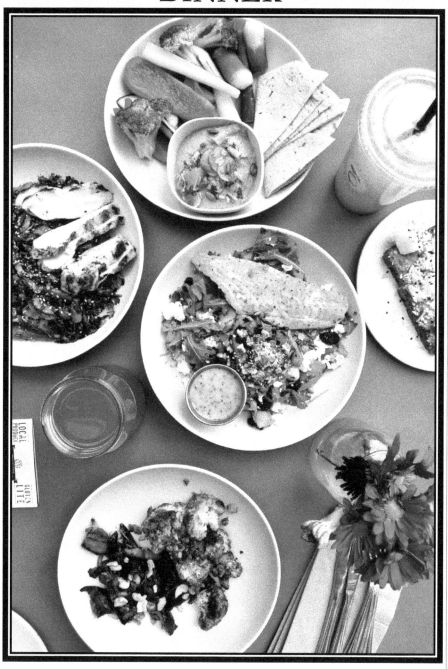

13. INDIAN CURRY WITH CAULIFLOWER

Directions time: 35 minutes
Servings: 4 servings
Difficulty level: Very easy

INGREDIENTS

- **400** G CAULIFLOWER
- **2** CARROTS
- **600** G CHICKEN BREAST FILLET
- **40** G BUTTER
- **2-3** TBSP CURRY POWDER
- **100** ML VEGETABLE STOCK (YEAST-FREE)
- **200** G CREAM

DIRECTIONS

1. Wash and clean the cauliflower and cut into small florets. Peel and slice the carrots. Cut the meat into large cubes. Heat the butter in a large saucepan and fry the chicken in it.
2. Stir in vegetables and curry powder and let simmer. Season to taste with salt and pepper. Gradually stir in the broth with the cream and let it simmer for 10 minutes.

VARIATION:
The fresh cauliflower can easily be exchanged for frozen cauliflower

Nutritional information
410 kcal; protein 39 g; fat 25 g; carbohydrates 8 g

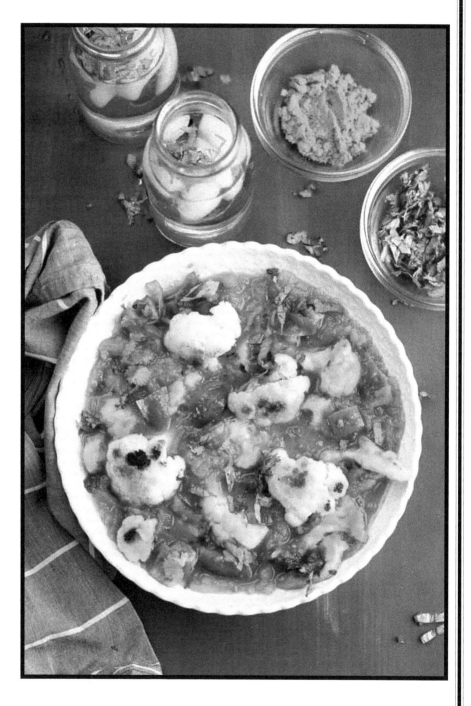

14. FENNEL AU GRATIN

Directions time: 25 minutes
Servings: 4 servings
Difficulty level: Very easy

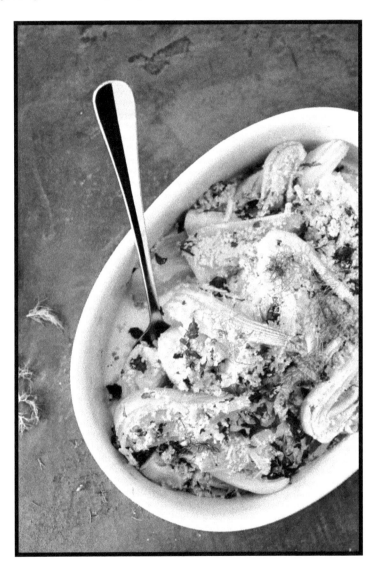

INGREDIENTS

- **800** G FENNEL
- **200** G CRÈME FRAÎCHE
- **100** G GRATED YOUNG GOUDA CHEESE
- **70** G PISTACHIOS OR OTHER
- WHOLESOME NUTS
- SALT
- PEPPER
- SOME BUTTER

DIRECTIONS

1. Wash off the fennel bulbs. Separate the fennel greens then chop them finely and set aside. Cut the tubers lengthways into 1 cm thick slices. Bring salted water to the boil and cook the fennel for about 3 minutes. Then allow the slices to drain thoroughly.

2. Brush a casserole dish with butter and lay out the fennel slices, slightly offset. Pour the crème fraîche into a bowl, add the cheese and pistachios and mix well.

3. Season with pepper. Distribute the crème fraîche evenly over the fennel and gratinate at 220 degrees (convection 200 degrees) on the middle rack until golden brown. Garnish with fennel green before serving.

VARIATION:

You can also prepare other vegetables such as carrots, onions or mushrooms in this way.

Nutritional information
420 kcal; protein 15 g; fat 36 g; carbohydrates 9 g

15. SESAME SALMON WITH PAK CHOI AND MUSHROOMS

Directions time: 30 minutes
Servings: 2 servings
Difficulty level: normal

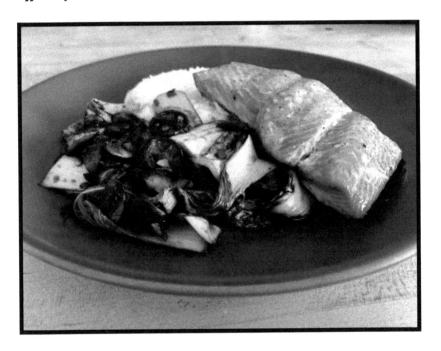

INGREDIENTS

- **300** G SALMON FILLET (FROZEN)
- **15** G SESAME SEEDS
- **250** G PAK CHOI
- **100** G MUSHROOMS
- **150** G KING OYSTER MUSHROOMS
- **1** HALF RED CHILI (IF COMPATIBLE)

- **1** CLOVE OF GARLIC
- **10** G GINGER
- **2 ½** TBSP SESAME OIL
- GROUND CORIANDER
- SALT
- SOME VINEGAR (IF COMPATIBLE)

DIRECTIONS

1. Thaw salmon quickly or use immediately. Roast the sesame in a pan until golden brown and bring the oven to 160 degrees (convection).

2. Cut the stems and leaves of the pak choi into strips and cut the mushrooms into bite-sized pieces. Finely chop the chili, garlic and ginger and briefly toss in sesame oil together with pak choi stems and mushrooms.

3. Add the pak choi leaves and let them collapse for a moment. Season to taste with coriander and salt and lay out in a casserole dish oiled with sesame oil.

4. Fry the salmon fillets briefly on all sides in the still hot pan, place on the vegetables and bake in the oven for about 8-10 minutes. Wet the salmon with a little vinegar and serve sprinkled with sesame seeds.

Nutritional information
392 kcal; protein 35 g; fat 28 g; carbohydrates 115 g

16. BELL PEPPER AND CABBAGE STEW WITH SAUSAGES

Directions time: 40 minutes
Servings: 4 servings
Difficulty level: Easy

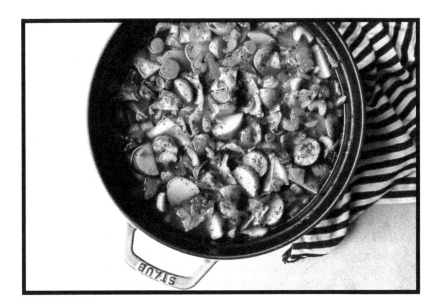

INGREDIENTS

- **2** RED ONIONS
- **1** CLOVE OF GARLIC
- **1** RED PEPPER
- **1** YELLOW PEPPER
- **450** G POINTED CABBAGE
- **300** G METTENDEN (FRESH OR FROZEN)
- **2** TBSP RAPESEED OIL
- PEPPER

- SALT
- **2** TBSP PAPRIKA PULP
- **700** ML BEEF STOCK
- **1** CAN OF CHUNKY PEPPERS
- **10** SMALL SNACK CUCUMBERS
- **2** SPRIGS OF PARSLEY
- **1** PINCH OF SUGAR
- **1** TBSP VINEGAR (IF COMPATIBLE)
- **4** TBSP CRÈME FRAÎCHE

DIRECTIONS

1. Peel the onions and cut into large cubes. Peel the garlic and chop very finely. Clean and wash the peppers and cut into pieces. Clean and wash the pointed cabbage, cut into two and remove the stalk. Cut the cabbage into strips approx. 1 cm wide. Cut the beef ends into slices.

2. Let the rapeseed oil get hot in a saucepan, sauté the garlic and onions until translucent. Add the cabbage and paprika and fry, turning constantly. Season to taste with salt and pepper. Add paprika pulp, sweat and pour over the beef stock and canned paprika. Bring to the boil and add the meatballs as an insert. Let the lid simmer for about 20 minutes.

3. In the meantime, cut the cucumber into large cubes. Put the cucumbers in the stew 5 minutes before the end of the cooking time.

4. Wash parsley, shake dry and finely chop. Season the stew with salt, pepper, sugar and vinegar. Serve with a dollop of crème fraîche and sprinkled with parsley.

Nutritional information
605 kcal; protein 24 g; fat 42 g; carbohydrates 39 g

17. MUSHROOM SOLYANKA

Directions time: 25 minutes
Servings: 4 servings
Difficulty level: Easy

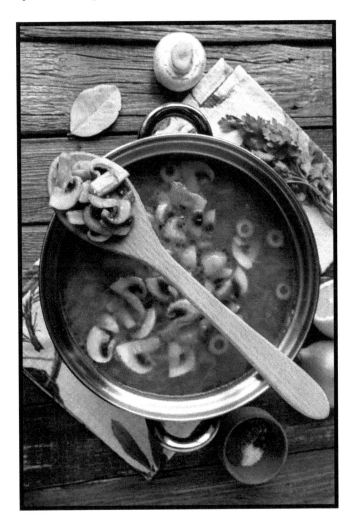

Nutritional information
112 kcal; protein 4 g; fat 9 g; carbohydrates 3 g

INGREDIENTS

- **250** G MUSHROOMS
- **800** ML WATER
- **1** BAY LEAF
- **3** ONIONS
- **3** CUCUMBERS
- **2** TBSP RAPESEED OIL
- **4** TBSP PAPRIKA PULP
- **10** OLIVES (ONLY IF TOLERATED)
- SALT
- PEPPER
- **3** STALKS OF DILL
- **4** TBSP SOUR CREAM

DIRECTIONS

1. Clean and wash mushrooms and cut into slices or cubes. Bring water to a boil in a saucepan, add a bay leaf to the water, add salt and simmer the mushrooms in it for 20 minutes.

2. In the meantime, peel and chop the onions. Wash cucumbers and cut into cubes.

3. Let a coated pan get hot, add rapeseed oil and sweat the onions in it until golden brown. Stir in cucumber and paprika pulp and simmer for about 5 minutes. Then add everything to the mushrooms and simmer for 10 minutes.

4. Pour olives into the soup and season with salt and pepper. Wash the dill, shake dry and chop into flags.

5. Divide the soup on four plates, put on 1 tablespoon of sour cream and serve garnished with dill.

18. BAKED PORK FILLET MEDALLIONS WITH APPLE

Directions time: 30 minutes
Servings: 4 servings
Difficulty level: normal

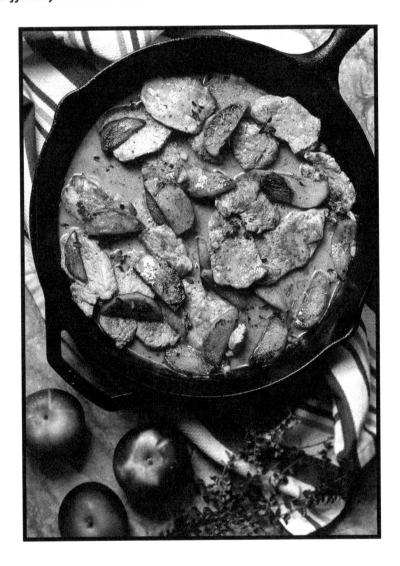

INGREDIENTS

- **1** RED ONION
- **1** RED APPLE
- SOME VINEGAR (IF COMPATIBLE)
- **600** G PORK TENDERLOIN
- SALT
- PEPPER
- **2** TBSP RAPESEED OIL
- **100** G SHEEP CHEESE OR FETA
- **2** STALKS OF MARJORAM

DIRECTIONS

1. Peel the onion and cut into wedges. Wash the apple, dry it well, cut it open and remove the core. Cut the apple into wedges and moisten with vinegar.

2. Wash the meat, pat dry and cut into four medallions of equal size. Top with salt and pepper.

3. Let the oil get hot in a pan. Fry medallions vigorously on all sides for about five minutes, turning, and remove from the pan.

4. Sweat the onion and apple in the hot frying oil. Season to taste with salt and pepper. Put medallions back in the pan. Crumble the cheese, spread over it and let it melt. Wash marjoram and shake dry. Remove the leaves and serve sprinkled over the medallions.

Nutritional information
220 kcal; protein 33 g; fat 8 g; carbohydrates 4 g

19. CHICKEN IN COCONUT SAUCE WITH SNOW PEAS

Directions time: 45 minutes
Servings: 3 servings
Difficulty level: normal

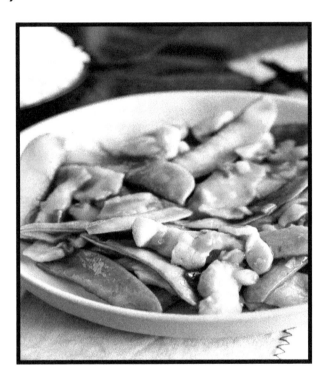

INGREDIENTS

- **500** G CHICKEN BREAST
- **150** G COCONUT MILK
- **250** ML VEGETABLE STOCK, INSTANT, YEAST-FREE
- **100** G YOGURT, LACTOSE-FREE
- **5** TBSP CREAM, LACTOSE-FREE

- **200** G SUGAR SNAP PEAS
- **15** G GINGER, FRESH
- **½** TSP TURMERIC
- **1** BUNCH OF CORIANDER GREENS, FRESH
- **½** SMALL SHALLOT
- SOME LEEK
- SOME RAPESEED OIL FOR FRYING
- SALT AND WHITE PEPPER
- PEPPERS

DIRECTIONS

1. Wash the chicken breast, pat dry and cut into small strips. Peel and chop the onion. Wash the vegetables, cut the leek into rings, peel the fresh ginger and cut into small cubes.

2. Fry the chicken breast lightly in oil, add the onion and fry, add a little pepper and pour in the broth. Stir in the coconut milk, add turmeric to taste. Add the leek, ginger and snow peas and let it boil down for about 20 minutes, stirring every now and then.

3. Add yoghurt and bring to the boil again. Take from the stove and chop the fresh coriander over it. Season to taste with salt and pepper. Rice tastes very good with it.

4. You can also add a little paprika and cook it briefly.

5. Those who tolerate it can also bring a little sharpness into the game. Since chili, or "spicy", often leads to problems with a histamine intolerance, you have to try carefully here.

Nutritional information
405 kcal; protein 13 g; fat 14 g; carbohydrates 41 g

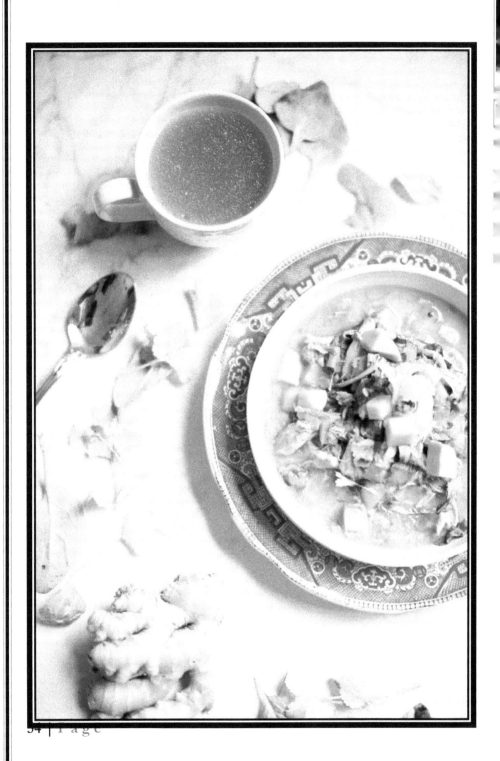

Snacks

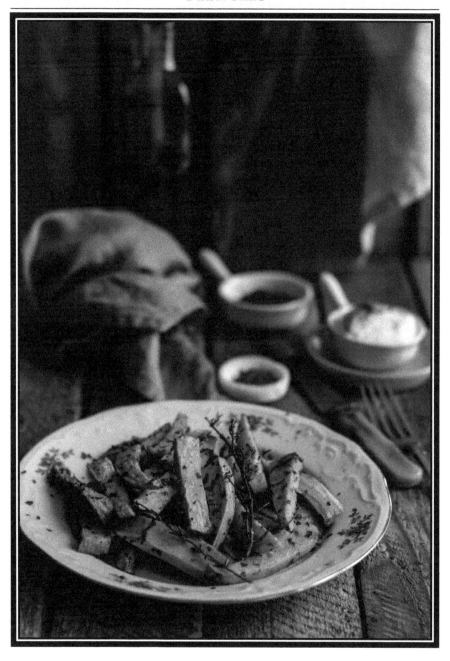

20. KOHLRABI IN SESAME CHEESE COATING

Directions time: 50 minutes
Servings: 4 servings
Difficulty level: Very easy

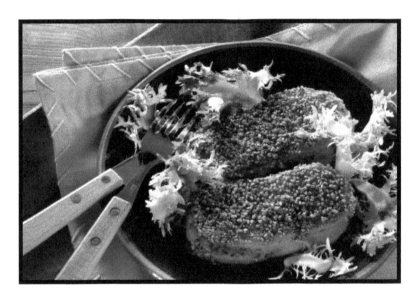

INGREDIENTS

- **800** G KOHLRABI
- **1** SHALLOTS
- **1** CLOVE OF GARLIC
- **½** BUNCH OF MINT
- **250** G MILD ORGANIC YOGURT
- **4** TBSP OLIVE OIL
- SALT
- PEPPER
- **2** EGGS

- **150** G SESAME SEEDS
- **100** G FRESHLY GRATED MOZZARELLA
- **50** G SPELLED FLOUR
- **100** ML THAI CHILI SAUCE (IF TOLERATED)
- CHILI FLAKES (IF TOLERATED)

DIRECTIONS

1. Clean the kohlrabi, peel off the skin, wash it and cut into long thick sticks. Pour into boiling salted water and cook for 5-6 minutes. Drain in a colander and let cool.

2. Peel the shallot and garlic. Cut the shallot into fine cubes and press the garlic through a garlic press. Wash the mint and remove the leaves from the stem. Set aside except for a few leaves for garnish. Cut the remaining leaves into fine strips.

3. Mix the yogurt, diced shallots, garlic and mint. Season with salt and pepper. Pour the yoghurt dip into a bowl and add olive oil. Open the egg in a deep plate and whisk with a little salt and pepper.

4. Mix the sesame seeds and grated mozzarella in another deep plate. Pour flour into a third plate. Roll the kohlrabi sticks in the flour, then in the egg and finally in the sesame mixture. Let the oil get hot in a pan and fry the kohlrabi in portions, turning until golden brown. Drain on kitchen paper and keep warm.

5. Serve together with the yogurt dip and the chili sauce. Garnish with mint and chili if you like and serve.

Nutritional information
330 kcal; protein 12 g; fat 22 g; carbohydrates 20 g

21. **FILLED PAPRIKA BITES**

Directions time: 20 minutes
Servings: 4 servings
Difficulty level: Very easy

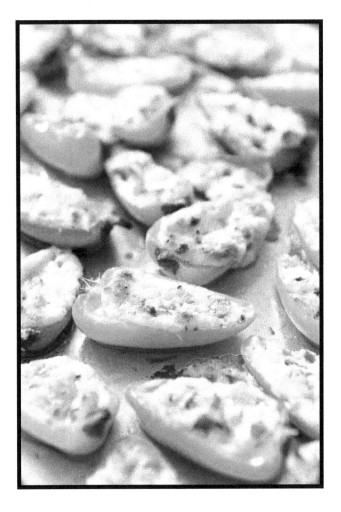

Nutritional information
260 kcal; protein 15 g; fat 14 g; carbohydrates 20 g

INGREDIENTS

- **70** G PAPRIKA PULP
- **50** ML OF WATER
- ½ TEASPOON OREGANO (DRIED)
- ½ TEASPOON BASIL (DRIED)
- PEPPER
- SALT
- **2** YELLOW PEPPERS
- **2** RED PEPPERS
- **2** GREEN PEPPERS
- **100** G CORN (CAN), IF COMPATIBLE
- **1** SHALLOT
- **100** G GRATED MOZZARELLA
- **100** G GRATED YOUNG GOUDA CHEESE
- **2** STALKS OF BASIL
- PEPPER, FRESHLY GROUND

DIRECTIONS

1. Mix the paprika pulp with water to a smooth sauce and season with oregano, basil, pepper and salt.
2. Wash the peppers thoroughly and cut lengthways into three parts. Remove the cores and partitions. Shed corn. Peel the shallot and cut into rings.
3. Bring the oven to temperature with 180 degrees top / bottom heat. Spread the paprika with the paprika sauce, put the cheese on top and cover with corn and shallots.
4. Place on a baking sheet lined with baking paper and bake in the oven for about 10 minutes.
5. Wash the basil, shake until dry, strip the leaves from the stem and cut into fine strips. Garnish the paprika pizza with basil and serve sprinkled with freshly ground pepper.

22. ZUCCHINI ENCHILADAS

Directions time: 45 minutes
Servings: 4 servings
Difficulty level: normal

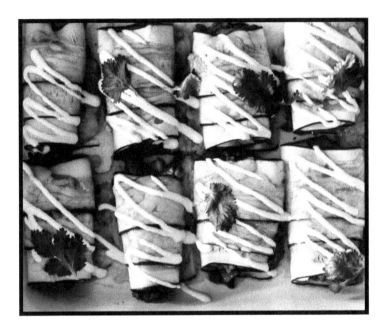

INGREDIENTS

- SOME FAT FOR THE SHAPE
- 1 RED ONION
- 2 CLOVES OF GARLIC
- 1 TBSP OLIVE OIL
- SALT
- 375 G CHICKEN, COOKED
- 1 TEASPOON CUMIN, GROUND
- 2 TEASPOONS OF CHILI POWDER, IF COMPATIBLE

- **150** ML TACO SAUCE, COMPATIBLE- ALTERNATIVELY PAPRIKA PULP
- **2** LARGE ZUCCHINI
- **100** G MOZZARELLA, GRATED
- **100** G GRATED GOUDA CHEESE
- **2** STALKS OF CORIANDER
- **100** G SOUR CREAM

DIRECTIONS

1. Bring the oven to 175 degrees and grease a baking dish (approx. 22 x 32 cm).

2. Peel and chopfinely the onion and garlic. Heat the oil in a pan and sweat the onions in it for about 5 minutes until golden brown. Salt. Chop the chicken into small pieces. Add the garlic, spices, chicken and 100 ml taco sauce, mix everything and cook for about 5 minutes over medium heat.

3. Wash the zucchini and cut lengthways into thin slices using a peeler. Lay out 5 slices next to each other on a board, slightly overlapping. Put 2 tablespoons of the filling on the lower end and roll the zucchini slices with the filling into a roll. Put in a baking dish. Prepare the remaining slices and filling as described.

4. Scatter 50 ml of taco sauce and both types of cheese on the enchiladas. Approx. Bake for 20 minutes.

5. Wash coriander, shake until dry and chop leaves. Take the enchiladas out of the oven and serve immediately garnished with sour cream and coriander.

Nutritional information
486 kcal; protein 39 g; fat 31 g; carbohydrates 15 g

23. **FILLED RICE BALLS WITH HAM & MOZZARELLA CHEESE**

Directions time: 210 minutes
Servings: 12 pieces
Difficulty level: normal

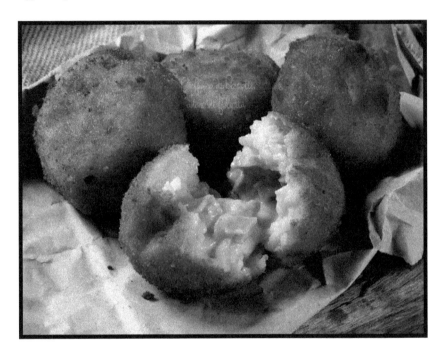

INGREDIENTS

- **1.2** LITERS OF WATER
- SALT
- **500** G RICE (ARBORIO OR VIALONE NANO)
- **1** SACHET OF SAFFRON (0.1 G)
- **30** G BUTTER
- **100** G GRATED YOUNG GOUDA CHEESE

- 30 G COOKED HAM
- 60 G MOZZARELLA
- 200 G FLOUR
- BREADCRUMBS
- VEGETABLE OIL FOR DEEP-FRYING

DIRECTIONS

1. Bring the water to a boil, add salt, put rice in boiling water. Halfway through the cooking time and stir in the saffron and cook the rice until cooked. When the rice is cooked all the water should have been absorbed by the rice. Mix the butter in pieces into the rice. Grate the Gouda cheese and stir it into the rice mixture. Then spread the rice in a flat bowl, cover with foil and let cool completely for at least two hours.

2. For the filling, cut the ham and mozzarella into small cubes.

3. Prepare a bowl with water (approx. 300 ml), slightly moisten your hands in it. Approx. 130 g of rice mass are required for each ball. Pour ⅔ of the mixture into the arch of one hand, press flat, then form a well in it. Fill this with some ham and mozzarella and seal with the rest of the rice. Then roll everything into an even ball.

4. When all the rice balls are ready, mix the flour with water to a smooth mass and prepare breadcrumbs. Dip the rice balls in the flour water then turn them in breadcrumbs. Let the vegetable oil get hot in a high saucepan and gradually fry the rice balls in it. Drain on kitchen paper and serve hot immediately.

Nutritional information
346 kcal; protein 10 g; fat 12 g; carbohydrates 48 g

24. KALE CHIPS WITH HERB DIP

Directions time: 55 minutes
Servings: 2 servings
Difficulty level: Very easy

INGREDIENTS

- **1** KG OF KALE
- OIL
- SALT
- **50** G HERBS OF YOUR CHOICE
- **150** G YOGURT (**3.5%** FAT)
- **1** TBSP OLIVE OIL
- **1** TEASPOON MEDIUM HOT MUSTARD
- **1** TEASPOON HONEY

DIRECTIONS

1. Firstly, wash the kale thoroughly until it is clean. Then remove the fine leaves from the stems and lay them out on some kitchen paper. In a large, deep saucepan, let the oil get hot (it will be hot enough if you hold a stick in it and blister it). Pluck the kale leaves to the desired size and fry them in the oil for about 2 minutes in several courses so that the whole leaves become crispy and look like chips. Drain on kitchen paper and add a little salt. Now lay out the chips on a baking sheet lined with baking paper and let them dry in the oven at 80 degrees with the oven door open for about 10 minutes.

2. Mix the herbs with the yoghurt, olive oil, mustard and a little honey, season with salt. Serve the dip with the kale chips.

Nutritional information
175 kcal; protein 11 g; fat 8 g; carbohydrates 7 g

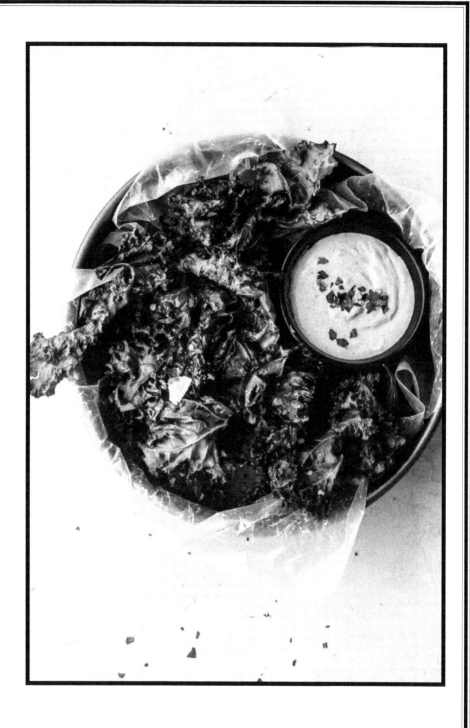

25. GRILLED CHEESE SANDWICH WITH PEACH AND BACON

Directions time: 20 minutes
Servings: 2 servings
Difficulty level: Very easy

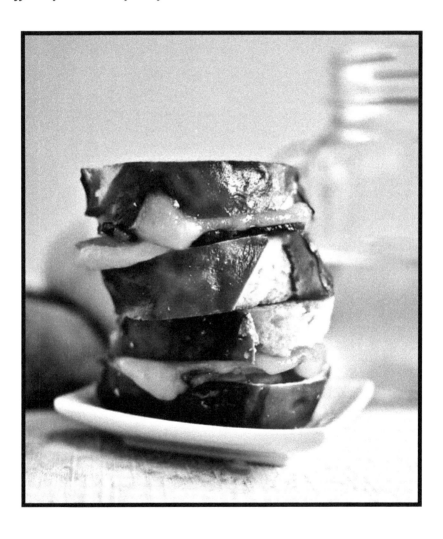

INGREDIENTS

- ½ RED ONION
- 100 G BACON (SLICES)
- 1 TEASPOON OF OIL
- 2 PEACHES (FRESH)
- 2 SLICES OF YOUNG GOUDA CHEESE
- 4 SLICES OF SAFE (TOAST) BREAD
- 2 TBSP BUTTER
- 4 TEASPOONS OF APRICOT JAM

DIRECTIONS

1. Peel the onion and cut into fine rings. Fry the bacon in a pan until crispy, then remove it from the pan. Let the oil get hot in the pan and sweat the onions until they are brown then remove them from the pan. Cut the peaches into small cubes. Split the gouda slices into two.

2. Butter each slice of bread on one side. Cover the other side with 1 teaspoon of apricot jam.

3. Place the peach cubes and onion rings on the jam and cover with half a slice of Gouda cheese. Place the bacon slices on top of the cheese and cover with another half slice of Gouda cheese. Place the second slices of bread on the sandwiches with the buttered side down.

4. Let a grill pan get hot and grill the sandwiches over low heat until the cheese melts. Press the sandwiches together with a spatula. Remove sandwiches from the pan, cut in two and serve hot.

Nutritional information
616 kcal; protein 21 g; fat 41 g; carbohydrates 44 g

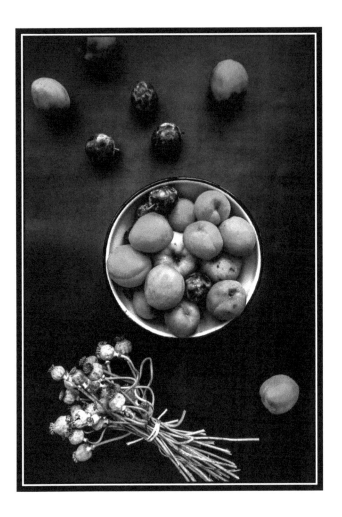

Dessert and Pastries

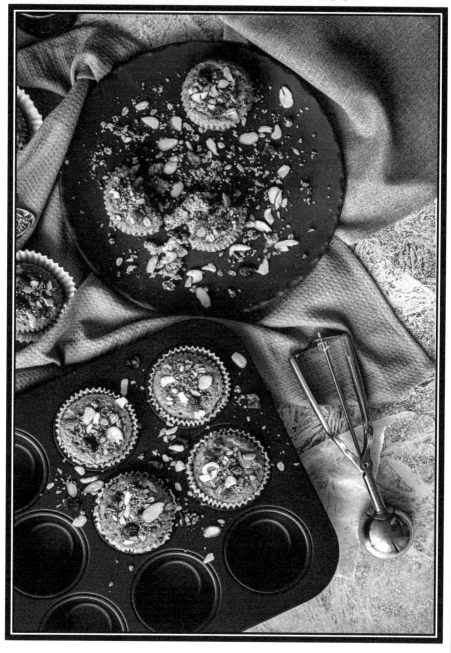

26. APRICOT CAKE

Directions time: 70 minutes
Servings: 12 pieces
Difficulty level: Easy

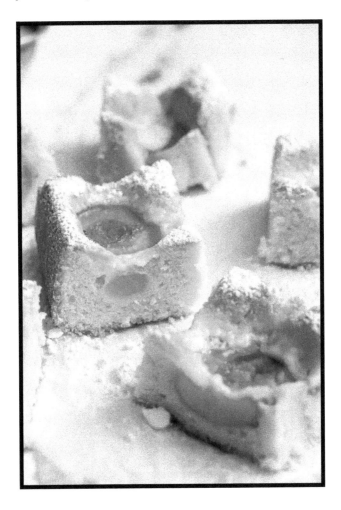

Nutritional information
147 kcal; protein 9 g; fat 12 g; carbohydrates 19 g

INGREDIENTS

- **100** G PECANS
- **150** G GROUND ALMONDS
- **3** EGGS
- **8** APRICOTS
- **3** TBSP FLEA SEEDS (ALTERNATIVELY
- CRUSHED FLAXSEED)
- **1** TBSP HONEY
- **1** TSP BAKING POWDER
- COCONUT OIL (FOR GREASING)

DIRECTIONS

1. Bring the oven to temperature with 180 degrees circulating air. Grease a springform pan thoroughly.

2. Put a few particularly beautiful nuts aside for decoration. Cut 3 apricots into thin slices for decoration. Chop the remaining pecans.

3. Use a hand blender to puree the remaining apricots together with the vanilla to a smooth mass.

4. Beat eggs and baking powder with a hand mixer and whisk until frothy. Add all other ingredients to the egg mixture and work in.

5. Pour the batter into the greased spring form pan. Decorate with nuts and apricot wedges.

6. Bake for about 50 minutes at 180 degrees on the middle rack. Take the cake out of the oven and let it cool down in the tin for 10 minutes. Then carefully remove the cake from the mold and then let it cool down completely. Dust with powdered sugar and serve with whipped cream.

27. **WHITE CHOCOLATE DREAM**

Directions time: 120 minutes
Servings: 12 pieces
Difficulty level: medium

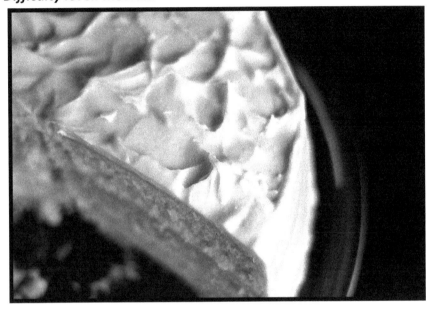

INGREDIENTS

- **190** G HAZELNUTS OR OTHER COMPATIBLE NUTS
- **30** G DESICCATED COCONUT
- **55** G COCONUT OIL
- **10** G COCOA POWDER (IF TOLERATED)
- **1** TEASPOON VANILLA POWDER
- **1** PINCH OF SALT
- **3** DATES (IF COMPATIBLE)

WHITE CHOCOLATE MASS :

- **100** G COCONUT OIL
- **30** G COCOA BUTTER
- **70** G SESAME MUSHROOMS (TAHINI)
- **55** G COCONUT MILK
- **2** TBSP HONEY
- **1** TEASPOON VANILLA POWDER
- **1** PINCH OF SALT

DIRECTIONS

1. Grind hazelnuts in a food processor. Add the remaining ingredients for the dark base and process until everything is well mixed and a kind of crumble dough can be seen.
1. Line the bottom of the cake pan with baking paper. Brush the edge with coconut oil. Pour the dark mixture into the cake tin then lay out evenly and press firmly.
2. Cover the cake tin with a little foil and place in the freezer.
3. In the meantime, beat all the ingredients for the white layer in the food processor or with the whisk of a hand mixer to a creamy mixture. Let the coconut oil and cocoa butter melt and then pull them into the creamy mass.
4. Spread the mixture on the already set base and place in the freezer for about 1 ½ hours until the mixture has set nicely.
5. To open the cake ring, let the cake thaw a little and carefully cut along the edge with a knife until the spring form pan can be easily removed.
6. Wet a sharp knife under hot water and carefully cut the cake into small pieces for serving.

Nutritional information
233 kcal; protein 8 g; fat 4 g; carbohydrates 31 g

28. NEW YORK CHEESECAKE WITH BLUEBERRIES

Directions time: 180 minutes
Servings: 12 pieces
Difficulty level: Easy

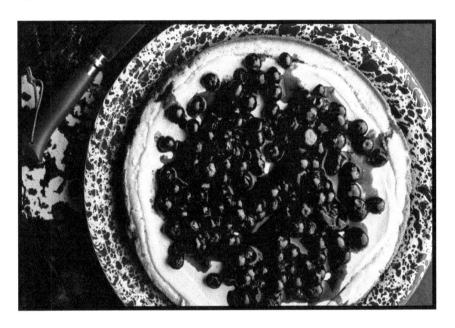

INGREDIENTS

- **120** G DESICCATED COCONUT
- **120** G HAZELNUTS OR OTHER WHOLESOME NUTS
- **4** TBSP COCOA POWDER (IF COMPATIBLE)
- **6** TBSP COCONUT OIL
- **2** TBSP HONEY
- **250** G COMPATIBLE NUTS

- **100** ML COCONUT MILK
- **200** G BLUEBERRIES
- **1** PINCH OF VANILLA

DIRECTIONS

1. Line the spring form cake tin with baking paper and grease the edge thoroughly.

2. Grind hazelnuts, desiccated coconut and cocoa powder in the food processor to form a kind of flour. Add 2 tablespoons of coconut oil and 1 tablespoon of honey until everything becomes uniform. Press the batter to the bottom of the spring form pan and place in the freezer.

3. Wash off compatible nuts and pour into the food processor with the coconut milk, the remaining coconut oil, honey and vanilla. Mix everything until the mixture is completely creamy.

4. Divide the mass and put half aside. Pour the other half onto the cake base and put the cake back in the freezer.

5. Put the other half of the cream in a food processor, add the blueberries and mix everything together well.

6. Spread the blueberry mixture on the cake, smooth out the mixture and put it back in the freezer.

7. Take out of the freezer and let thaw 1 hour before serving. Cut open the cake with a knife heated under hot water and serve immediately.

Nutritional information
154 kcal; protein 8 g; fat 8 g; carbohydrates 19 g

29. GINGER BREAD MOUSSE

Directions time: 15 minutes
Servings: 2 servings
Difficulty level: medium

INGREDIENTS

- **200** G PRE-COOKED CHESTNUTS
- **1** EGG YOLK
- **2** TBSP HONEY
- **150** ML COCONUT MILK
- **1** PINCH OF CINNAMON
- **1** PINCH OF GROUND CLOVES
- **1** PINCH OF GROUND NUTMEG
- **1** PINCH OF GROUND CORIANDER

DIRECTIONS

1. Heat chestnuts and coconut milk in a saucepan over medium heat. Then puree until smooth with the hand blender. Depending on the desired consistency, add coconut milk to the mixture.

2. Add honey and spices to the mixture then turn off the stove.

3. Finally stir in the egg yolks and let them set while stirring constantly. Divide the dessert into dessert bowls and place in the refrigerator until ready to serve.

Nutritional information
372 kcal; protein 4 g; fat 20 g; carbohydrates 40 g

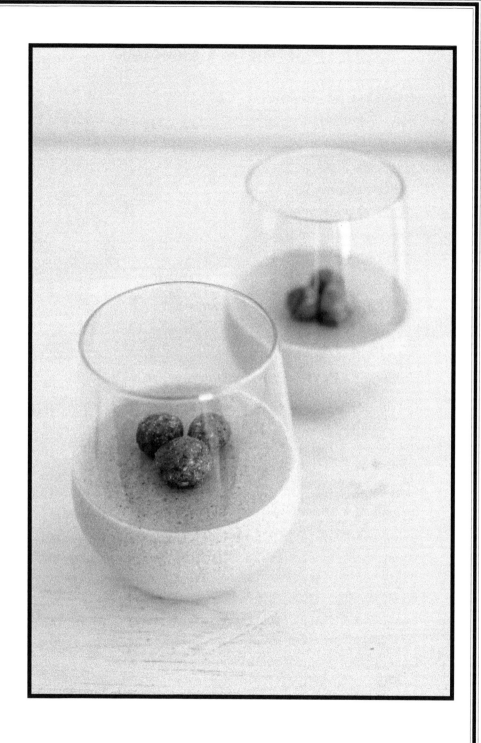

30. PUMPKIN COOKIES

Directions time: 80 minutes
Servings: 20 cookies
Difficulty level: Easy

INGREDIENTS

- **100** G PUMPKIN SEEDS
- **100** G CASSAVA FLOUR
- **20** G ARROWROOT STARCH
- **2** TBSP HONEY
- **100** G BUTTER
- **50** G WHITE CHOCOLATE, IF COMPATIBLE

DIRECTIONS

1. Grind the pumpkin seeds into flour in the food processor. Mix with cassava flour and arrowroot flour.

2. Cut butter into pieces and add honey. Knead into a ball of dough together with the flour from the food processor, alternatively knead with your hands to form a smooth ball of dough.

3. Shape the dough into a roll (about 3-4 cm in diameter) and place in the refrigerator to rest for half an hour.

4. Bring the oven to 160 degrees Celsius and line a baking sheet with baking paper. Take the dough out of the fridge, cut the biscuits off the rolling pin and place them on the baking sheet.

5. Bake in the oven for 12 minutes. Cover half of the completely cooled biscuits with melted chocolate. If you have intolerance, leave out the chocolate.

Nutritional information
68 kcal; protein 4 g; fat 1 g; carbohydrates 13 g

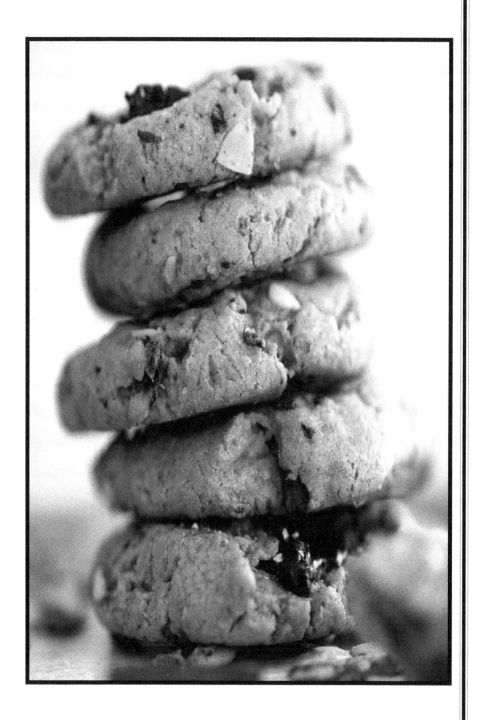

31. BEETROOT JELLY

Directions time: 40 minutes
Serving: 3
Difficulty level: Medium

INGREDIENTS

- **1** CAN **BEETROOT**
- **1** PACKET **PORT WINE JELLY**
- **500** GMS **HOT** WATER
- **SQUIRT** CANOLA SPRAY

DIRECTIONS

1. Boil water and melt jelly crystals.
2. Spray a glass pie dish.
3. Drain the rest of the beetroot juice into the jelly and mix through.
4. Layer the beetroot on the bottom of the pie dish covering the bottom of the dish. Pour the jelly over the beetroot.
5. Cover and refrigerate until set. Cut up into squares.

Nutritional information
8 kcal; protein 0 g; fat 0 g; carbohydrates 2 g

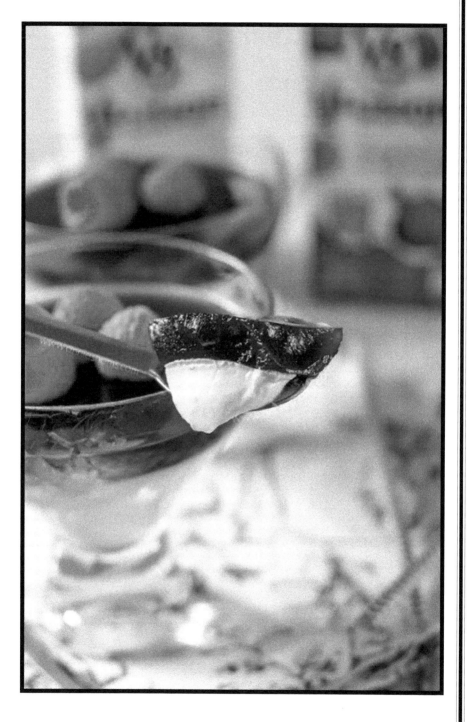

32. BAKED APPLE

Directions time: 40 minutes
Servings: 3 servings
Difficulty level: Very easy

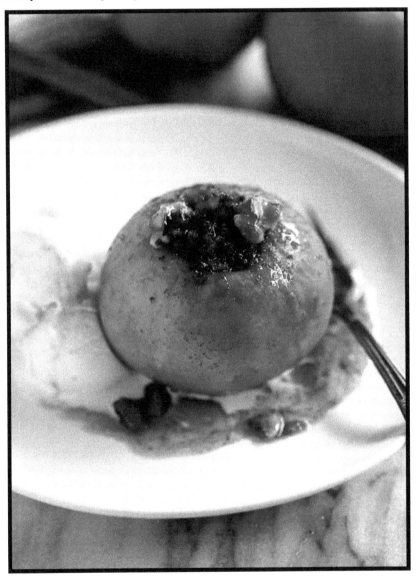

INGREDIENTS

- **3 GRANNY SMITH APPLES** (OR DEPENDING ON YOUR PREFERENCE)
- **50** G GROUND ALMONDS
- **10** G CINNAMON (MORE IF YOU LIKE)
- **3** TBSP HONEY
- **2** TBSP BUTTER (MELTED)
- **60** G RAISINS (OR CRANBERRIES), DEPENDING ON TOLERANCE
- **50** G HAZELNUTS OR OTHER NUTS, DEPENDING ON TOLERANCE

DIRECTIONS

1. Cut off about the upper eighth of the apples with a sharp knife (including the stem). Then carefully remove the casing with the knife without destroying the lower end of the apple.

2. Mix the almond flour, cinnamon, honey and melted butter in a saucepan. Mix in the raisins and finely chopped hazelnuts.

3. Then fill the baked apple with the mixture with a teaspoon and carefully stuff it so that the apple is well filled.

4. Preheat the oven to 150 degrees and bake the baked apples for about 30 minutes.

Nutritional information
307 kcal; protein 4 g; fat 15 g; carbohydrates 40 g

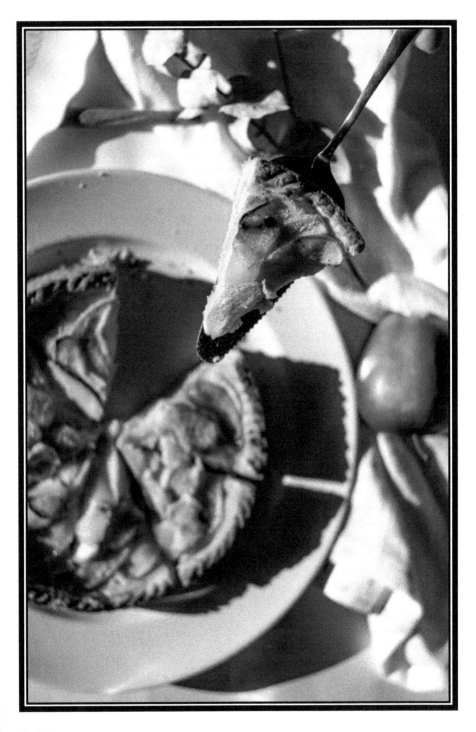

Soups

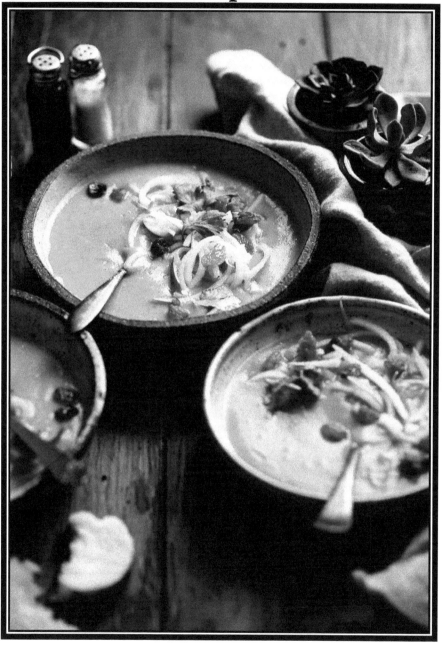

33. ASPARAGUS SOUP

Directions time: 15 minutes
Servings: 2 servings
Difficulty level: Easy

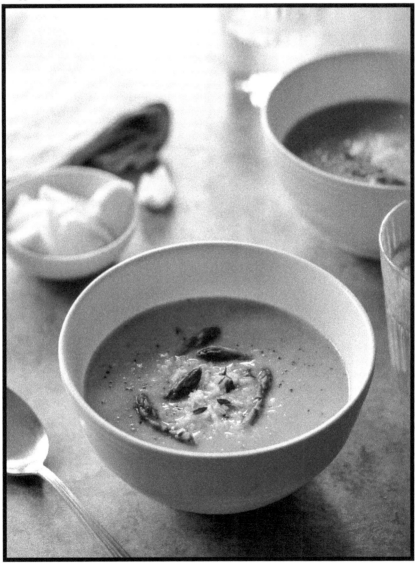

INGREDIENTS

- **50** G BUTTER
- **1** PINCH OF SALT
- **1** RED ONION
- **1** CLOVE OF GARLIC
- **1** BUNCH OF WHITE ASPARAGUS
- **500** ML WATER / BROTH
- **1** PINCH OF NUTMEG
- **1** DASH OF VINEGAR (IF TOLERATED)
- **2** SPRING ONIONS (OPTIONAL)

DIRECTIONS

1. Peel off the skin of the onions and garlic and chop or cut both very finely.

2. Melt the butter in a small saucepan and sweat the onion and garlic pieces in it until translucent. Add a little salt.

3. Separate the woody ends of the asparagus remove the skin from the asparagus and then cut into pieces.

4. Put the asparagus in the pot and sweat it, then pour water or broth over the whole thing.

5. After 15 minutes, puree the soup with a hand blender to the desired consistency; pass through a sieve to taste and season with nutmeg, vinegar and salt. Arrange the soup with spring onions and serve hot.

Nutritional information
74 kcal; protein 2 g; fat 2 g; carbohydrates 4 g

34. CELERY SOUP

Directions time: 25 minutes
Servings: 2 servings
Difficulty level: Easy

INGREDIENTS

- **1** CELERY ROOT
- **1** CLOVE OF GARLIC
- **1** RED ONION
- **2** TABLESPOONS OF LARD OR BUTTER
- **200** ML COCONUT MILK
- **100** ML OF WATER
- **1** PINCH OF VANILLA, GROUND
- **1** PINCH OF NUTMEG, GRATED
- **1** PINCH OF SEA SALT

DIRECTIONS

1. Peel the peel of the celery root and roughly chop the celery. Also, peel off the peel of the onion and garlic and chop both.
2. Melt the fat in a saucepan and sweat the vegetables in it until they have turned a little color. Add salt immediately after frying.
3. Then add the coconut milk and water and let it boil until soft.
4. Finally puree the soup with a hand blender to the desired consistency and season with the spices. Serve the soup hot!

Nutritional information
272 kcal; protein 13 g; fat 19 g; carbohydrates 9 g

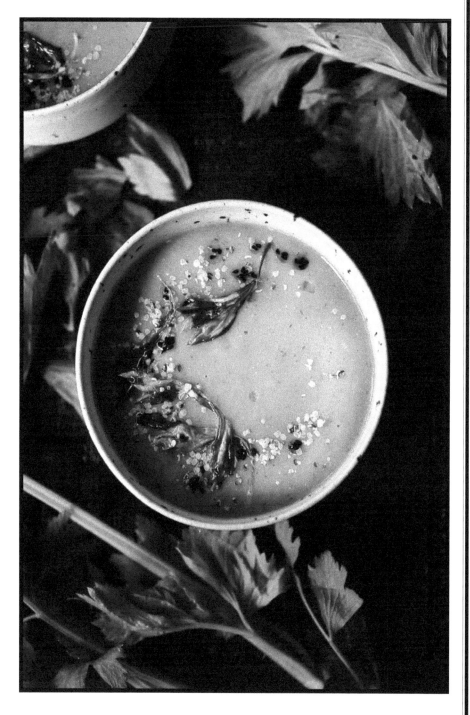

35. BELL PEPPER SOUP WITH MEATBALLS

Directions time: 55 minutes
Servings: 3 servings
Difficulty level: Easy

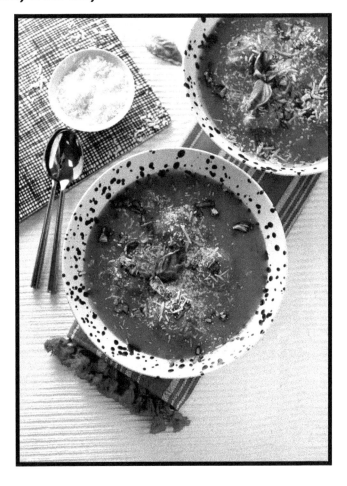

Nutritional information
148 kcal; protein 16 g; fat 23 g; carbohydrates 8 g

INGREDIENTS

- **3** RED PEPPERS (ABOUT **600** G)
- **1** RED ONION
- **1** CLOVE OF GARLIC
- ½ RED CHILI (IF TOLERATED)
- **1** TBSP OLIVE OIL
- **1** LITER OF BROTH
- **1** PINCH OF SALT AND PEPPER
- **1** SPRING ONION
- **300** G GROUND BEEF (FRESH AND SELF-MINCED)
- **1** EGG YOLK
- **2** TEASPOONS OF MUSTARD
- **1** TEASPOON PAPRIKA PULP
- **1** TBSP COCONUT OIL

DIRECTIONS

1. Wash the peppers, remove the seeds and partitions and cut everything into cubes. Peel the onion and garlic and roughly chop. Wash and chop the chili too.

2. Let the olive oil get hot in a saucepan. Sweat the paprika, onion, garlic and chili in it. Pour in the vegetable stock and cook covered for about 15 minutes. Puree the soup with a hand blender until the consistency you want and season with salt and pepper.

3. While the soup is cooking, prepare the meatballs. To do this, wash and finely chop the spring onions.

4. Knead a meat dough from minced meat, spring onion, egg yolk, mustard and paprika pulp. Refine with salt and pepper. Shape the meat dough into about 12 balls. Fry in hot coconut oil on all sides in a pan for about 5 minutes. Then add the meatballs to the previously pureed soup and let them steep for 10 minutes. Then enjoy the soup hot.

36. MOROCCAN SOUP

Directions time: 30 minutes
Servings: 2 servings
Difficulty level: Easy

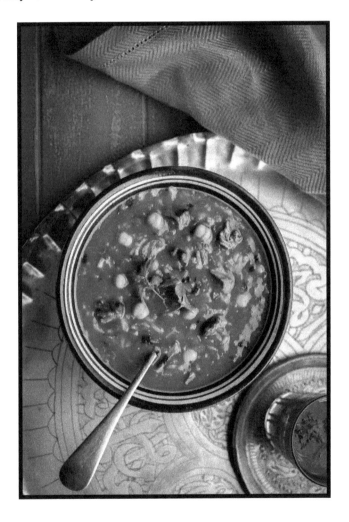

Nutritional information
267 kcal; protein 13 g; fat 18 g; carbohydrates 23 g

INGREDIENTS

- **500** G SWEET POTATOES
- **2** CARROTS
- **1** RED ONION
- **2** CLOVES OF GARLIC
- **1** TBSP BUTTER
- **400** ML OF BROTH
- **100** ML COCONUT MILK
- **1** TEASPOON PAPRIKA POWDER
- **½** TSP CHILI
- **1** PINCH OF CUMIN
- **1** PINCH OF NUTMEG
- **½** TEASPOON SALT
- **1** PINCH OF PEPPER
- SOME VINEGAR (IF COMPATIBLE)
- FRESH CORIANDER AS A GARNISH

DIRECTIONS

1. Peel the skin of the sweet potato and carrot and cut into large pieces.
2. Cut the onion and garlic into cubes.
3. Let the butter get hot in a tall saucepan. Fry the onions, garlic, sweet potatoes, and carrots in it for about 5 minutes.
4. Pour the broth over the top and let it simmer over a medium heat for about 10 minutes.
5. Stir the coconut milk and spices into the soup and cook for another 5 minutes.
6. Once the vegetables have been cooked and the soup can be pureed to the desired consistency with a hand blender.
7. Serve the soup with chopped coriander and serve while it is still hot.

37. KOHLRABI STEW

Directions time: 30 minutes
Servings: 4 servings
Difficulty level: Very easy

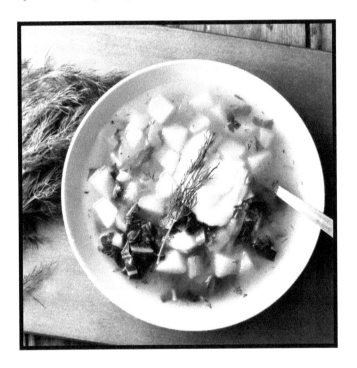

INGREDIENTS

- **1** RED ONION
- **2** LARGE KOHLRABI
- **2** CARROTS
- **2** FLOURY POTATOES
- **1** TBSP BUTTER
- **2** BAY LEAVES
- **3** JUNIPER BERRIES
- **5** WHOLE PEPPER CORNS

- **1** BUNCH OF FRESH PARSLEY
- **500** ML OF BROTH
- **1** TEASPOON SALT

DIRECTIONS

1. Peel the onion and cut into fine cubes.
2. Peel the peel of the kohlrabi and carrots and cut into bite-sized pieces.
3. Peel the skin of the potatoes as well and roughly grate them in a bowl using a kitchen grater.
4. Let the butter get hot in a large saucepan. Sauté the onion, kohlrabi, carrots, bay leaves, juniper berries, peppercorns and parsley for about 2-3 minutes.
5. Pour in the broth and add the grated potatoes to the soup. The soup is bound by the floury-boiling potatoes and no additional flour is required.
6. The vegetables should also be covered with the broth. If necessary, a little water can be added if the broth boils down too quickly.
7. Now bring the soup to the boil for about 20 minutes on a medium heat with the saucepan covered. Stir through the soup from time to time so that nothing burns.
8. When the vegetables are done but still slightly firm to the bite, season with salt.
9. Remove the bay leaves and juniper berries from the soup, garnish with fresh parsley and serve hot.

Nutritional information
110 kcal; protein 6 g; fat 5 g; carbohydrates 12 g

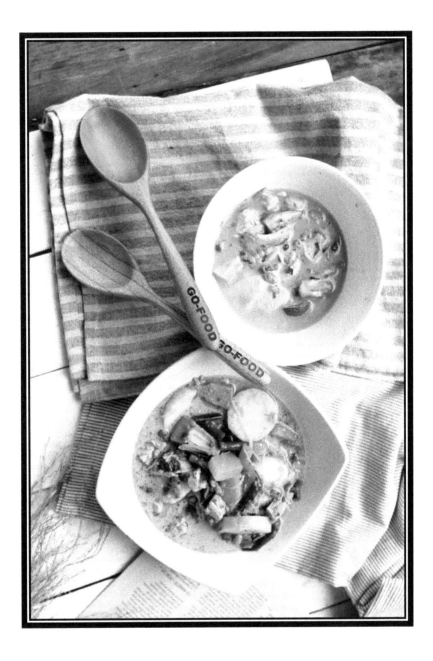

Salads

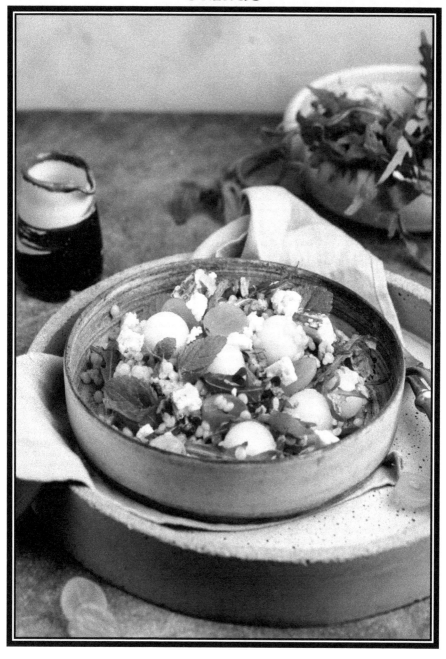

38. WILD HERBS SALAD

Directions time: 10 mins
Servings: 2 servings
Difficulty level: Easy

INGREDIENTS

- 2 HANDFULS OF WILD HERBS (LADY 'S MANTLE, QUENDEL, CHICKWEED , CLOVER, GROUND ELDER, RIBWORT, NETTLE, BEDSTRAW, NASTURTIUM, DANDELION, BLOOD VESSEL)
- 4 RIPE PLUMS
- 1 HANDFUL OF RED CABBAGE
- 1 SPRING ONION

FOR THE DRESSING:

- 3 TBSP OLIVE OIL
- 2 TBSP VINEGAR (IF TOLERATED)
- 50 G BLUEBERRIES
- 1 TBSP HONEY

DIRECTIONS

1. Wash the collected wild herbs well and spin dry using a salad spinner. Then roughly chop with a large knife. Wash the plums, remove the stone and cut the plums into eight parts. Cut the red cabbage and the spring onion into fine strips. Collect all ingredients in a salad bowl.

2. For the dressing, whisk all ingredients in a stand mixer to a creamy sauce and, depending on the consistency desired, add a little water. Season with salt and pepper. Mix the salad with the dressing just before serving and serve immediately so that it does not collapse.

Nutritional information
144 kcal; protein 5 g; fat 7 g; carbohydrates 8 g

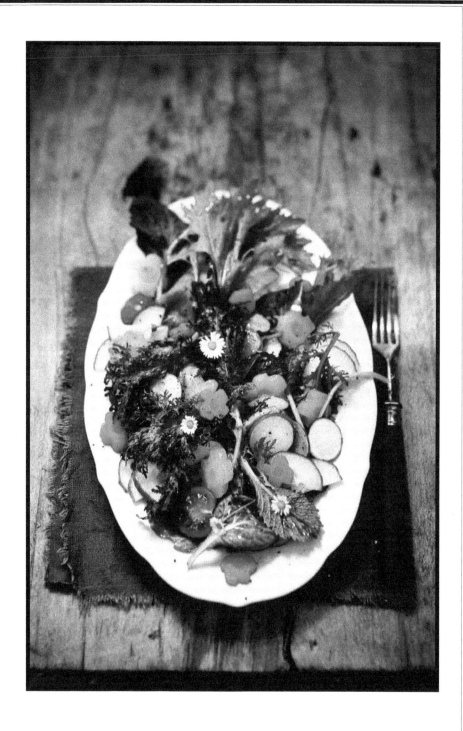

39. BROCCOLI AND CARROT SALAD

Directions time: 25 minutes
Servings: 2 servings
Difficulty level: Easy

INGREDIENTS

- **1** BROCCOLI
- **5** CARROTS
- ½ ICEBERG LETTUCE
- **3** TBSP SESAME SEEDS
- **2** TBSP APPLE CIDER VINEGAR (IF COMPATIBLE)
- **3** TBSP OLIVE OIL
- **1** TEASPOON MUSTARD
- **1** CLOVE OF GARLIC
- **1** TEASPOON THYME
- **1** PINCH OF SALT, PEPPER

DIRECTIONS

1. Cut broccoli into small florets and cook in salted water until al dente. Peel the skin of the carrots and grate in the food processor (alternatively with the kitchen grater).
2. Cut the iceberg lettuce into bite-sized strips. Mix the lettuce, broccoli and carrots together in a bowl. Take the garlic out of the shell and press.
3. Whisk together a dressing made from garlic, mustard, oil, apple cider vinegar, thyme, salt and pepper.
4. Pour the dressing and sesame seeds over the salad just before serving.

Nutritional information
126 kcal; protein 4 g; fat 10 g; carbohydrates 9 g

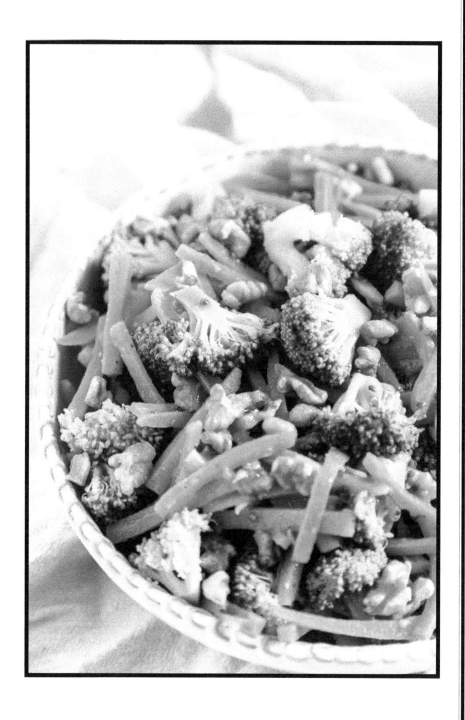

40. WARM PARSNIP SALAD

Directions time: 35 minutes
Servings: 2 servings
Difficulty level: Easy

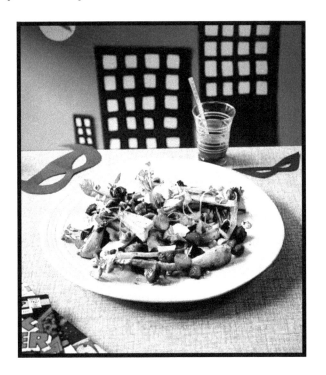

INGREDIENTS

- **400** G PARSNIPS
- **250** G CHESTNUTS (PRE-COOKED)
- **2** TBSP OLIVE OIL
- **2** TBSP ROSEMARY CHOPPED
- **2** HANDFULS OF FRESH SWISS CHARD
- **1** SPRING ONION

FOR THE DRESSING:

- **1** TEASPOON HONEY
- **2** TBSP APPLE CIDER VINEGAR
- (IF COMPATIBLE)
- **2** TBSP OLIVE OIL
- **4** TBSP APPLE JUICE (IF TOLERATED)
- **1** PINCH OF SALT
- **1** PINCH OF PEPPER

DIRECTIONS

1. Bring the oven to a temperature of 200 degrees.
2. Peel the skin of the parsnips and dice the parsnips. Mix with olive oil and chopped rosemary and season with a little salt and pepper.
3. Also, cut the pre-cooked chestnuts into cubes and mix with the olive oil and rosemary.
4. Spread the parsnips on a baking sheet and bake for 20 minutes. Halfway through, add the chestnuts to the parsnips in the oven.
5. While the parsnips and chestnuts are baking in the oven, wash the chard and distribute on plates. Cut the spring onion into fine rings and sprinkle over the chard.
6. Mix the dressing and pour over the salad.
7. At the end, sprinkle the roasted parsnips and chestnuts over the salad and serve the salad warm.

Nutritional information
424 kcal; protein 219 g; fat 19 g; carbohydrates 39 g

41. KOHLRABI SALAD

Directions time: 10 mins
Servings: 2 servings
Difficulty level: Easy

INGREDIENTS

- **2** KOHLRABI
- **1** LARGE TART APPLE
- A COUPLE OF MINT LEAVES

FOR THE DRESSING:

- **2** TBSP OLIVE OIL
- SOME VINEGAR (IF TOLERATED)
- **1** TEASPOON MUSTARD
- **1** TEASPOON HONEY
- ½ TEASPOON SALT
- **1** PINCH OF PEPPER

DIRECTIONS

1. Remove the peel from the kohlrabi. Peel the peel of the apple and roughly grate the kohlrabi and apple or cut into pieces of your choice.
2. Wash the mint leaves, shake until dry and finely chop.
3. For the dressing, whisk all ingredients together well.
4. Mix everything together, let it steep a little before serving and then enjoy the salad.

Nutritional information
Kcal 114 kcal; protein 1 g; fat 8 g; carbohydrates 9 g

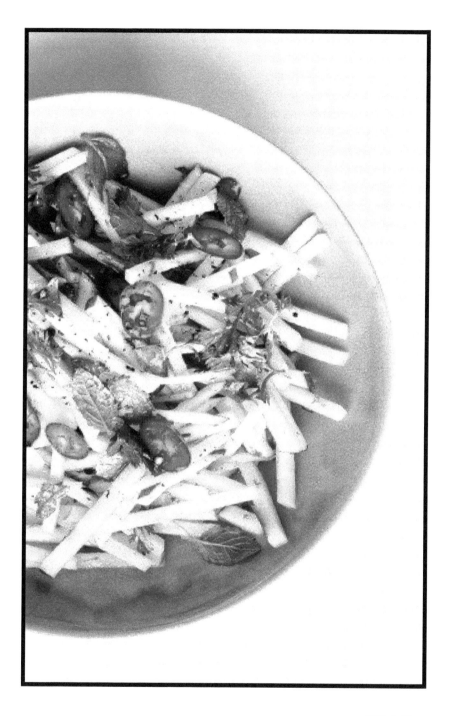

42. PAK CHOI SALAD

Directions time: 15 minutes
Servings: 2 servings
Difficulty level: Easy

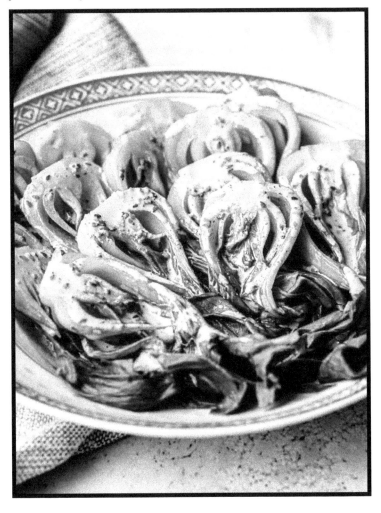

Nutritional information
304 kcal; protein 1 g; fat 33 g; carbohydrates 4 g

INGREDIENTS

- **2 PAK CHOI**
- **1** HANDFUL OF GREEN SALAD
- **1** STALK OF CELERY
- **2** SPRING ONIONS
- **1** HANDFUL OF FRESH HERBS (BASIL, PARSLEY, MINT)
- **100** G HAZELNUTS OR OTHER WHOLESOME NUTS

FOR THE DRESSING:

- **4** TBSP OLIVE OIL
- **½** TEASPOON VINEGAR (IF COMPATIBLE)
- **1** TEASPOON HONEY
- **1** TEASPOON MUSTARD
- **1** PINCH OF SALT
- **1** PINCH OF PEPPER

DIRECTIONS

1. For the dressing, whisk all the ingredients together, season to taste and, if necessary, add seasoning.

2. For the salad, wash the pak choi and the green salad thoroughly and cut or pick into bite-sized pieces. Thoroughly wash and clean the celery stalk and cut into bite-sized pieces.

3. Wash the spring onions thoroughly and cut into fine rings. Wash the herbs, spin until dry and roughly chop.

4. Mix the salad vegetables with the dressing and sprinkle the hazelnuts whole or chopped over the salad as a crispy topping. Serve the salad immediately!

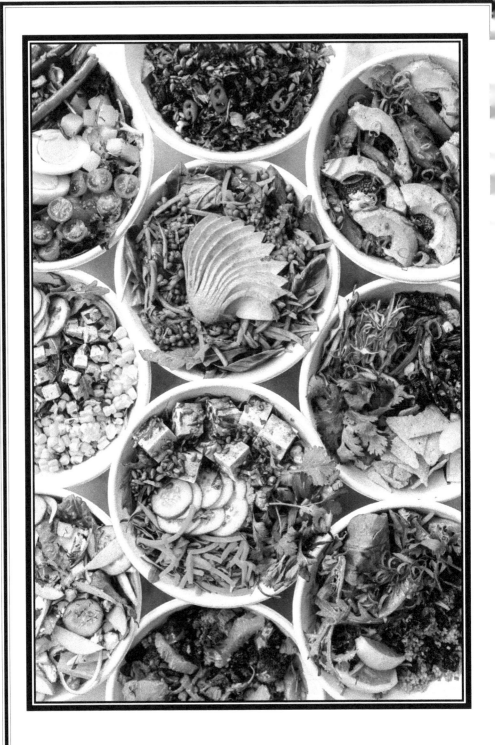

CONCLUSION

Of course, the primary aim of the nutrition plan is to help you feel good and enjoy your prepared food without regrets but you won't win anything if you consume too many calories on a regular basis. In the end, the food is digestible, but it is reflected on the hips. Therefore, you should determine your daily calorie requirement. How does this work? First, calculate your basal metabolic rate using the following formula:

WOMAN

(Body weight in kilograms x 10) + (height with in centimeters x 6.25) - (age x 5) - 161

MAN

(Body weight in kilograms x 10) + (height in centimeters x 6.25) - (age x 5) + 5

The calculated calorie requirement then of course also takes your daily activity into account. The corresponding factor, which is then multiplied with the equation above, is calculated equally for men and women as follows:

- 1.20 Not at all active , sedentary work and if activities, then a maximum of 1 x per week

- 1.37 A bit active , sedentary work, if active, then once or twice a week

- 1.55 Quite active , regular physical activity, light physical work

- 1.72 Very active , sport or very physical work almost every day

- 1.90 The professional sector , at least 2 times a day sports and especially physical activities at work

DO YOU WANT TO LOSE WEIGHT, BUILD MUSCLE OR STICK TO YOUR WEIGHT?

This is also taken into account in the nutrition plan:

- To Lose weight = 300 kcal are deducted from the calculated result
- Hold = It remains with the calculated result
- Muscle building = 300 kcal are added to the calculated result

Here I would like to show you a calculation example for a woman and a man:

1. **Woman, 73 kg, 168 cm, 39 years old, a bit active, goal: to keep weight**

$\{(10 \times 73) + (6.25 \times 168) - (5 \times 39) - 161\} \times 1.37 = (730 + 1050 - 195 - 161) \times 1.37 = 1424 \times 1.37 = 1951$ kcal

So, with this calculation you can take in 1951 kcal per day while maintaining your weight.

2. **Man, 72 kg, 182 cm, 35 years old, very active, goal: keeping weight**

- $\{(10 \times 72) + (6.25 \times 182) - (5 \times 35) + 5\} \times 1.72 = (720 + 1138 - 175 + 5) \times 1.72 = 1688 \times 1.72 = 2903$ kcal

So, the daily calorie consumption in this example is thus 2903 kcal per day.

In this way, you can calculate your personal calorie requirement.

Cooking and preparing low histamine meals and dishes cannot be compared to dieting! After all, when you ingest foods that are not good for you, you will feel a good amount of suffering, and you will not even be happy if you cook and prepare only foods and dishes that you do not tolerate.

But wellness also happens on the plate.

You don't have to give up anything, but this point is not easy: many will immediately agree, especially on the tomato point. After all, very few people with histamine intolerance can tolerate this vegetable, although exceptions can confirm the rule. While everyone around you eats tomato pasta with gusto, you should not be chewing on your lettuce leaf. Of course, a good salad can be delicious; however, from the moment you feel you have to give it up, you become miserable.

This situation may not happen the first time, but sooner or later, it will happen.

So I ask you to prepare your happiness on your plate as well! It may look more elaborate, and some dishes may even have deviations, but it doesn't make them any less tasty.

Just because something has been listed as unsafe or indigestible doesn't mean you can't tolerate it at all. Of course, it can happen that you can't let certain foods, after all; otherwise, you wouldn't suffer from histamine intolerance, but again I'd like to take the example of yeast.

A surprising number of people with histamine intolerance can tolerate even small amounts of yeast quite well. Therefore, you don't necessarily have to give up fluffy, light Sunday sandwiches. Instead, bake them yourself and see how they take to you. Find your intolerance by doing small trials, slowly and without forcing too much.

If you really can't tolerate that food, you can replace it with something else. For example, you can replace yeast with baking powder! A bolognese does not always have to be made with ground meat and packaged tomatoes! The same goes for applesauce: anyone can buy it, but homemade is still much better!

Over time, you'll get a feel for the foods that are good for you and the ones that make your life difficult. You will get to know yourself better and adjust your food preferences accordingly. You may not be able to enjoy tomatoes with mozzarella cheese, but mushrooms sautéed in garlic or parsnip chips with peach chutney will! Life can be delicious when you know how to do it. I wish you more wellness and always enjoy a bit of culinary happiness and many culinary moments at the same time.

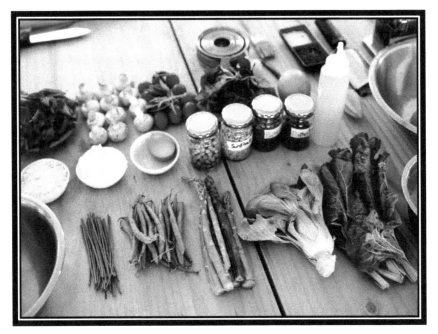

CPSIA information can be obtained
at www.ICGtesting.com
Printed in the USA
BVHW051945151021
619042BV00010B/174